Lift it High

Copyright © 2023 by Brigitte Adofo Agyapong

All Rights Reserved. No part of this publication may be reproduced, stored in a retrieval system or transmitted in any form or by any means electronic, mechanical, photocopying, recording, scanning or otherwise, except by permission from the author.

ISBN: 978 – 9988 – 3 – 5943 – 0

For enquiries, contact the author on

Address: P. O. Box AF 3124, Adenta
Email: contactus@brigitteaagyapongwrites.com
Tel: +233 (0) 545 322 615

Designed and Printed by

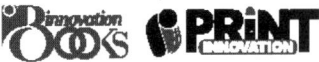

+233 (0) 267 771 670
+233 (0) 572 007 000
www.print-innovation.com
www.innovationbooks.net

Disclaimer

Although this book is designed to provide accurate information with regard to the subject matter covered, the publisher and the author assume no responsibility for errors, inaccuracies, omissions or any other inconsistencies herein.

This book is meant as a motivational or inspirational guide to help readers achieve their dreams. However, it is not meant as a replacement for direct expert assistance. If such level of assistance is required, the services of a competent professional are to be sought.

For bulk purchases of the physical copies of this book or collections of my books, kindly send an email to discounts@brigitteaagyapongwrites.com

To invite Brigitte Adofo Agyapong to speak at your virtual or in-person events, kindly send an email to speaking@brigitteaagyapongwrites.com

RELATED BOOKS WRITTEN BY THE AUTHOR

Win You: An Introspective Journey Of Finding Yourself, Knowing Your Potentials And Harnessing Them For Greater Heights And Ultimate Success

The Search Workbook: 8 Master Keys To Unfold Life`S Purpose And Achieve Its Desired Success And Meaning

RELATED JOURNALS

Goal Setter and Implementer Journal
Mood Tracking Journal
Emotional Mastery Journal
Emotional Release Journal

Introduction	xiii
Live for your purpose	1
Where do you want to be?	5
C'mon craft those dreams	8
Be You	11
Always remember your light can make the foggy road clear	14
Shine everywhere	17
Move higher into the light	20
Never stop	23
Reflect on your today and Move	26
Learn and correct the mistake	29
Do something everyday	32
Fuel your mind with YOU	34
Establish values and ethics	37
Develop your daily Mantra	39
Throw out the negativity	41
Begin the Journey	43
Open up your senses	45
Visualize all images	47
Build these images into ideas	50
Start Planning	53
Start working	56
Believe in your dreams	59

Buckle up, arise and keep the fire burning	61
Develop an inspiration booster	65
Influence others too	68
The life is here	71
Pack the worry away	73
Nothing is impossible	75
Remove Doubt from your being	77
Give life a fresh start, there is nothing wrong when you fail	80
Build relationship with others	82
Take a break	86
Surround yourself with People who will support your dreams	88
Start journaling	91
The passion is yours, use it	95
Love yourself	97
Appreciate these steps	100
Be grateful	102
You Stopped your passion!	104
Just smile	107
The complains is enough, stop!	109
Give yourself the chance to grow	111
Be firm on your decision	115
Open up your ears, heart for advice	117
Life is a journey not a race	119
See challenges as a step to victory	122

Share love too	124
Be flexible	127
Set goals	129
Be open don't harbour pain in you	133
Add Prayer too	136
Develop a step Model to Succeed	138
Clinched yourself to other professionals	142
Learn to ask questions	145
Take risks	149
Think Big	153
Set Discipline Straight, Build boundaries around yourself	155
Wrap up: Dream bigger and higher	158
Note to you, my dear reader.	160
Bibliographies	162
Value added segment	164
Other Books	167

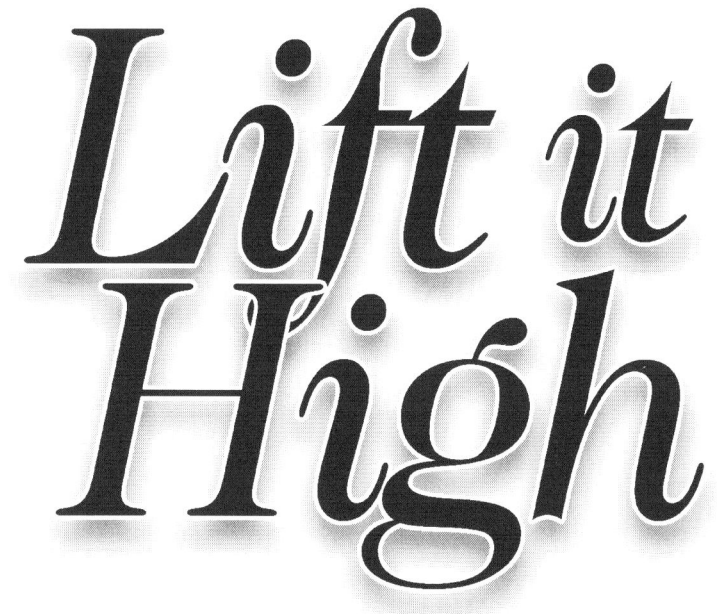

58 MOTIVATIONAL MESSAGES TO UPLIFT YOUR DREAMS INTO REALITY FOR THE DESIRABLE RESULTS INTO GREATNESS AND ELEVATION.

BRIGITTE ADOFO AGYAPONG

Acknowledgement

All thanks to Almighty God for the knowledge and wisdom to produce this book. Great! Another masterpiece has been completed to impact nations and transform generations.

I wouldn't have done this all by myself, in fact, I had a backbone supporting my dreams and this masterpiece.

To my accountability partners, Coach Rosie and Ebenezer Anane, thanks for every support towards my brand. All my advisors and supporters of my brand; Coach Rosie, Ebenezer Anane, Sophia Nkrumah, Portia Dwomoh, Reginald Nnuabue, Pastor Ayorka, Pastor Samuel Boateng and the Family; Bishop Benalvin Bennet, Mrs. Bertha Owusu, Mr. Samuel Ofosu Okyere, and all my loved ones who supported the brand, Brigitte A Agyapong. Thank You. I appreciate your effort.

To Nandani Rathore, Serwat Faisal, Rosie Kendall and the rest of my fans around the world who through your testimonials, assisted me in the concept of the idea of this book to help readers around the world. Thank You so much. I appreciate every word you sent across just to keep on going with what I do.

To all fans around the world, just to mention a few, fans in Ghana, USA, India, Uk, Canada, Germany, Brazil, Spain, Australia, Mexico, and the Philippines, your support is appreciated. You always support any initiative I bring out. Thank You.

And to all my members of the Launch team, John Otu, Enock Mensah, Corporal Richard Ngissah, Mumuni Chena Mohammed, Nelson Kofi Yeboah and Dzifa Tamakloe, thank you so much. I appreciate every effort you added to make this book a success.

Introduction

Do you want to achieve your dreams? How eager are you to achieve them? How hard are you working to reach where you want to be with your dreams? Do you sometimes get stuck when you are performing them? Have you ever thought of giving up on these dreams? If the major answers to these questions are yes, then you have picked the perfect book to suit your dreams.

As humans, we can get bored with the things we do and are subject to change. Sometimes, you feel reluctant to pursue these wonderful dreams which you started previously with high energy and eagerness. You have always said to yourself "no one can persuade me to give up." You felt on top of your life. You worked and continued to work with happiness, with the hope to see the dream fully progress, it started showing good results, but suddenly, challenges struck you, and it hit you hard that you couldn't imagine you wanted to give up. You felt like stopping because you didn't want to touch and work on it again.

Have you ever experienced this? Sometimes you may develop a new dream, but anytime you want to start working on it, a series of thoughts enter your mind, and these thoughts always try to bring in a negative energy to possess you. Speaking of ideas, you sometimes sprout thoughts and ideas which will ruin your dreams. You are in the state of the "fear factor." You fear to lose, fear to fail, fear to love, fear to start, and are covered by other touches of fear and negative emotions fighting back at you with a simple thought in your mind.

What I am eager to inform you about now is the energy to push you up when you feel like stopping or repudiating the dreams out of your DNA. Definitely, you will feel this in one way or another. Let me introduce to you what you need. You need a mental booster or an inspiration to boost you to rekindle your energy to keep on going. We lurk on this. We need the inspiration to pursue harder.

I encountered this idea after publishing my debut book, 'Win You', and started receiving direct messages through my social media handles and email on how the book is helping people to realize their potentials. Some of the messages brought my mind to the idea of writing this book purposefully to persuade, encourage, inspire and elevate you to continue working on your dreams, and surely one day, it will yield results. This book will back us with the high energy to build and yield our results to greatness. This book is here to inspire you to continue the wonderful dreams you want to embark on.

It will serve as a companion in times of struggle and will give you hope to try again until you get it right and win. Another motive for this book 'Lift It High', is to serve as a guide to direct your path to greatness.

How will you use it?

- This book can be used as a daily message to empower your day. You only need a ready mind willing to tap into the messages from this book to inspire you to work on your dreams.

- Utilize the activities in the book in the activities section.
- Share with others too because when you share the message with others, you have impacted thousand.

Enjoy and Impact.

Brigitte Adofo Agyapong

The discovery and definition of purpose is best enough to lead you in the journey of life

- Brigitte Adofo Agyapong

Live for your purpose.

Live with purpose everywhere. If you have found purpose, great! Big congratulations to you. Are you still working in line with your purpose? It is time to work according to it. If you are in the second group in which you know nothing about your purpose, something is tickling you to go for it. Are you eager to discover it? Good, the most important thing is that you have the desire and the willpower to go for it.

Don't worry, you have chosen the right book to suit your needs.

Finding purpose means finding your path and direction in life. It always keeps you and rekindles your energy to face the realities of life. Whether good or bad, purpose needs to be accomplished. With purpose, you know when to start, stop, pause, and continue on the endeavour you are embarking on. Even when the blow of life hits you hard, you are certain that this is where I want to go and love that even in challenges and struggles. Personally, I do love adventure movies; seeing people go on a far journey outside their comfort zones to seek treasurers to help in their research, out of curiosity, or save the community. I am always excited when I see people embark on such journeys in movies to save humanity. Most of these journeys are neither smooth nor rough but are faced with rough experiences most of the time, making people lose their lives in the process. Sometimes, their path becomes challenging as they experience problems in discovering paths to success, but never give up because they know their focus and the direction they are heading. And no matter what, they have to achieve their purpose, thus, to search for treasures that can save their society. They slip, fall, rise and walk, and run until they see treasures in their own hands, and then bring them back to benefit their society.

I guess you are thinking "O, this is a movie". I want to tell you this, though these are regular scenes from adventure movies. Life itself is an adventure, and to find the treasures in it, you need to find your purpose, and there are quite a number of experiences you will encounter in your life adventure. You will experience the bad, the ugly, the sweet, the bitter, the fall and the rise, all in search of a purpose. Some can find their purpose through a very bad encounter, whiles others find theirs in good experiences. In any way you find your purpose, whether good or bad, the vital point is that purpose has been discovered and found, and now you are working with it. Late Dr. Chadwick Bossman (May his soul rest in peace), once said that he found his purpose when he was experiencing cancer in his life, leading him to follow his purpose, and through his purpose, he landed into movie roles that gave him absolute peace of mind. Whilst battling cancer, he was still shooting movies. This particular message that he said at the Howard University commencement Speech really touched my heart and pushed me. It says sometimes you need to get knocked down before you can figure out what your fight is. Sometimes you need to feel the pain and sting of defeat to activate the real passion and purpose that God has predestined inside of you.

I don't want you to just say I have found my purpose without working according to it. Just finding and not flowing with your purpose is meaningless. When you find your purpose and live for it every day and everywhere, you feel the communication with yourself and the inner being, that a transformation has implemented in your life. In fact, the purpose energy you feel inside you becomes so strong that you will want to help others which you think can bring you inner peace, and when you do that, the feeling empowers you to do more. What is your purpose? Discover your purpose. It can be anything around you. Discover it. Don't let anyone tell you that this is your purpose or that is your purpose. Introspectively assess yourself, your needs, your identity, and everything about yourself.

Resources are available on the resources page for the discovery of purpose and the guidelines to follow to find yours. These books are, 'Win You: An introspective Journey of finding yourself, knowing your potentials and harnessing them for greater heights and ultimate success', and another book , 'The search workbook: (8 Master keys to unfold life`s purpose and achieve its desired success and meaning).'

Learn to live for your purpose. If you can discover your purpose, learn to work with it each time. Don't stop living, work with it because the more you live for it, the more you share the impact with the people around you, and in the end, you will receive absolute peace of mind and total happiness.

Purpose doesn't make life easy. It makes life possible.

– Dr. Myles Munroe

Where do you want to be?

You have beautiful dreams and nice aspirations. This message is to help you examine yourself on your wants, likes, hates and where you want to be. It becomes difficult to fully assess yourself and know your way when you are surrounded by things which make you fall prey to comparison, blame and copy, especially when you see your peers, friends, and other circles in your network succeeding up and up on the success ladder. You see them as people who have achieved their purpose whilst you dawdle behind. You have not succeeded as you wish, which renders you a 'prey' to the blame and copy desire. You now set dreams and goals which are far different from what you want and your purpose in life. You may pay less attention to the inner communication of your being. You neglect yours and rather focus on the dreams of others.

Now, it's time to focus on your purpose and your aspirations. You can assess yourself in these:

How far would you like to go with these dreams?

Where do you want to reach? Who would you like to impact or inspire?

Where do you want to be in the next years? At what pace do you want to go?

I have a dream, and you have yours, but for this dream to become reality, you will need to know how the dream is going to take off. Is this dream going to place you among the world's top 10 billionaires? Where do you want to go?

Is this dream going to help you to be called the world's fastest machine creator? Where do you want to go? And how far are you going? Is it fast or slow? Do you want to be a problem solver?

Do you know what you want? Go for it. Don't let any other noise distract you from working on yourself.

Pursue these wonderful dreams. I can't wait to see you on the top of the ladder of elevation. Go for it. You can do it.

The future belongs to those who believe in the beauty of their dreams.

–Eleanor Roosevelt

C'mon craft those dreams.

Why the wait? You have beautiful dreams leading to great aspirations. I don't think we should undermine one's dreams against the other. What is stopping you from realizing these dreams? I know your heart yearns for these great dreams. You have big and small aspirations of where you want to be in the next ten or twenty years. You hear from friends what they wish for in life. What they want to achieve in their lives in a countable number of years. Whenever you hear of these dreams, they become appealing to your ears and heart too. Hey, those dreams are big and great, can I create one too? Yes, you can, and you will create one, bigger and greater than the ones you hear. These questions of self-doubt were some of the questions I previously asked myself when I heard and saw that dreams come into reality. It was very admiring to me until I realized that I can. I can also create dreams too. My Wish can be created.

There is nothing special between someone who writes dreams and the other who doesn't. The truth is that dream is a wish. A wish for greatness, a wish for new initiatives and many more aspirations for one's life. The most important thing is that, with dreams, you can sit down and set your goals to accomplish those dreams. You can plan and create systems to make them work. They are beautiful and nice when you create them.

Crafting your dreams is simple. They are strong when you craft them. Crafting those dreams means you have strongly moved a step ahead to set goals and plan for your future. Dreams need to be critically planned. Don't just be open to people's thoughts in a way that you will emulate their style and dreams because they look beautiful to you. Have a sit in your room, pick a journal or a notebook, think quietly and assess what you really want in life and where you hope to be in designated years to come. Be yourself. Create those dreams, love the dreams you have created and move forward to build them up because dreams without action or end activities are mere wishes. They are void and can vanish in thin air. Working on those dreams means the hope to be this and that has come to stay and have a mark to be looked upon. Anytime you are working on your dreams, it reminds you and creates confidence in you that truly your dreams are achievable no matter what. Start Now.

Be yourself, don't take anything from and never let them take you alive.

– Gerard Way

Be You.

Be you in all your dealings. Everyone is unique in their own way. The earth has a great population of 7.9 billion spreading to every part of the seven continents and islands. Each one of the 7.9 billion population has an identity; likes, dislikes, behaviours, attitude and habit which forms his/her way of life.

Though our behaviour might be similar to one another, they can never be the same. Each one of us has our likes, dislikes, interest area, and much more which relate to our identity. Each one of us is unique. Our competencies are unique as much as our failures.

Can you imagine comparing your failure with someone's success? Do you know the in-depth success step pursued? How he or she did it? The in-depth of every action that led to the success? There is a big difference in that.

Even if you use the same approach in doing what a successful person did, there will be a slight difference in what empowered the person to the successful ladder, so as a failure. Never compare your failure to someone else's failure because you are two distinct individuals with competencies and flaws.

Love the advantages and disadvantages of your identity. Don't criticise and blame yourself for the imbalances you see in yourself and around you. Just love who you are because you have all the power in you to succeed in life. Everything is possible if you believe in the power in you and your words. Instead of comparing yourself with friends, family, colleagues and other people in your society, can you try this? Why don't you take a step forward to be yourself? Just try it. Accept the beauty of your identity even if you hate them, and challenge yourself on this.

Just be yourself. You are a unique and special person filled with excellence in everything you do. Even in your mistakes, you are unique! Show yourself the care and love which is needed to raise you in whatever endeavour you are willing to engage yourself in. Be you.

Let's do this. (Kindly put your name in the blank space, and proclaim positively).

I_____ believe that I am powerful and filled with excellence, and I love the real me.

You can also try an affirmation that works perfectly for you.

Your light can make the foggy road clear

- Brigitte Adofo Agyapong

Always remember your light can make the foggy road clear.

Wondering about this? What foggy road is the book talking about?

The road of life is neither smooth nor rough, we enjoy a mixture of both. The reality of life tells and allows us to learn that things can change at any time. Any direction we take has consequences; when you take the bad road, you enjoy your benefit likewise the good. The state of life is not all about the nature of the road, as muddy roads, a road filled with potholes, or smooth roads. You can be found on a muddy road but has a good or smooth road ahead. Life is a journey, and how you move can guide you to the successful end of it.

The foggy roads are the challenges we face when we try our best to achieve our dreams. Some setbacks push us to stop or pause whatever we are doing or wherever we want to go or reach. You can't see clearly on a foggy road unless you use a powerful or strong headlight or light to guide you to the clearer road where you are going.

This journey is likewise an encounter I had:

I quite remember years ago in Aburi, a town in the Eastern region of Ghana. I travelled to a town around the Akwapim-range which is a mountainous area. We travelled from Mamfe to Aburi around 4:30 am GMT. As we travelled, the road was foggy, so the driver could not see clearly. He switched on the headlight so that the bus could safely pass through the foggy road to a clearer road under the mountain. Instead of the normal speed, he drove slowly. Also, since the road was constructed on a mountain and was curvy as well, he took his time to drive slowly, and finally, the travellers arrived on a clear road.

Everyone experiences foggy roads; these encounters are just to stop us or convince us that our journey or any aspirations of ours are impossible. The foggy encounter can be people around us, problems causing setbacks, lack of emotional support for our dreams, financial constraint and many more. We sometimes become confused when we are even on the right track and faced with challenges. Don't let those foggy roads stop you, but rather, see them as step-stones which is giving you the strength to push through until you reach the clear road. Do you know you can do this? Yes, You can do it.

The light is the energy level you have inside of you which supports the dreams into reality even if you feel like giving up on the beautiful journey. Raise your willpower high and increase the momentum to push further, though it will take time. One step at a time; don't rush the process, and slowly, you will reach there with every step you take. Don't allow other distractions to affect your steps or moves, and let the energy rise to the top and be your lead. Don't slip, and even if you slip, consider that more height needs to be achieved. You are powerful, and you will rise. I really like this quote in 'Things Fall Apart' by Chinua Achebe; "The downfall of a man is not the end of his life." Push hard and walk again. Let the will to do more be at the blossom of your mind and heart until you bypass the trials and the problems.

Just keep going.

Stars don't shine because they want to be seen; they shine because they are stars.

- Alexander Den Heijer

Shine everywhere.

You are a star, there is a great need to shine everywhere. "I am facing a huge loss in business, how can I shine?"

You can shine perfectly even when you are stuck with challenges and problems in life. This is the right time to increase your energy level and be determined in whatever you do. Increase the booster inside you and work towards your goals. Thus, to change circumstances in and around your life. "No, I can't do it." Yes! you can, and you will do it. Motivate yourself.

When do stars shine? They shine in the dark so that you can see their beauty and splendour in the night. When you lift your eyes to the sky in the night, you see galaxies of stars forming together. They are beautiful. In all the darkness surrounding the stars, they can bloom and showcase their beauty, their strength, and competence.

Don't let the situations you are facing now stop you from moving out in line with your goals and aspirations. Be for it. Increase the inspiration to motivate and push yourself to go further. Relax, and don't think about the effect these problems are causing in your life. Be yourself, be strong and keep on going. Failing on these paths or steps means other steps need to be initiated to pave the way. Move one step and another step, Keep on going.

Do great in darkness, but don't forget to shine in the light also. Be strong for yourself. The more you allow yourself to shine, it then becomes your form and habit. Your mind will know you as a person who shines everywhere, and the society will also define you as the person whose state is to shine. You always gleam daily.

Keep the beauty up and shine.

> *Move into the light, there are no two ways about it. The more your light takes a step in darkness, the more darkness and challenges are reduced. Continue to move, and move stronger into the light and broaden your possibilities.*
>
> – Brigitte Adofo Agyapong

Move higher into the light.

You will surely reach there when you move. The energy, the grit, the power, and a lot more are in store for you and are all available in your hands.

I realised that, when you craft your dreams, set goals, and start working on them day by day, you achieve those goals. When you discover that you are on the edge of achieving your prioritised dream, you then hope for another wish which is more than the one you have achieved. As you grow, your needs and goals also expand. You yearn for more.

Creating another dream means you are advancing to another priority filled with challenges and problems. Get ready for the battle. It is good to give yourself more challenging tasks.

Don't stop yourself from creating and setting goals for a new horizon. Do it. Broaden your spectrum of capabilities and capacities. Move into success, and success is never a one-day affair. You rise, fall and rise, fall, slip and a whole lot on this journey. Allowing the problems ahead is normal and a plus for winning in life because it is part of the encounter. Move higher to a big destination of success. Keep on going. You will meet people who will support you and people who will disgrace you. Embrace those that support you and be vigilant against those that disgrace you; some indirectly show you the way and give you the strength to push forward. You will encounter big wins and small wins, but in all, appreciate whatever comes your way and live with it. Since you are moving higher, priorities, competencies and challenges will also be greater. Just open up to every encounter and critically assess them to know about each step you take. Move.

You can't win if you don't try

- Robin Sharma

Never stop.

Never stop going where you want to go. It is very okay when you pause on chasing what you want. There is a vast difference between pausing and stopping.

In both encounters, there is a cease in action to continue. One has greater momentum than the other. When you start a journey and you pause to rest, it means you want to gather some water or food to gain momentum to continue with the journey. The water or food can be related to the booster or inspiration to keep you going.

Though people around might perceive that you have stopped, instinctively, you know you just paused to rest. You paused to gather some courage and study all the possible risks, opportunities, and competencies to continue moving. With this action, you are preparing your mind to continue and start again. Since you have gathered all the necessary activities which include the competencies, power and energy to move and continue what you started, you become more energized than the former. More powerful than ever because you now know your strength and weakness, especially when you learn from your past mistakes to push through when circumstances similar to the previous ones take place. You can strongly rise and fight to move and keep going.

Keep on going, don't stop. When you stop chasing your dreams, it means you have quit and want to turn away from them.

When others are running, don't be confused and say "why am I not running fast as them? It takes time and purpose to reach where you want to go. Just keep walking. Since you are also moving, positive results will show in their time. Just move.

When I heard the story of Usain Bolt using 4 years of training to become the world's fastest man, thus, training for 4 years to win 9 seconds track record to take the title, I marvelled. Wow! That is it, never stop. If he had stopped, I don't think he would have reached where he is now. When you mention Usain Bolt, most of us know who he is. I call this; grit backed with power to pursue until you reach there. Are you still thinking about whether to continue? Don't stop. You can pause but remember to continue and persevere to where you want to go. See you at the top.

Great leaders develop through a never-ending process of self-study, self-reflection, education, training, and experience.

- Tony Buon

Reflect on your today and Move.

There are new beginnings every morning. New day, new moments. Why today? The most important thing is that you have the energy today, and you are pursuing life as it is today and not yesterday.

Blaming yourself on past events, I believe is meaningless because there is nothing in existence for it again. It only reminds you of the pain of "why did this happen to me?" When you do that, you stop yourself from thinking about how you can solve the problem. Previously, when I wasn't mature in the personal development phase of my mindset, when something bad happens to me, I do complain a lot and tried to blame others or myself. The usual phrase I query is "Why me? or Why must this happen to me? I realized that anytime this thought echoes in my head, it does this to me instead; it increases the pain of the encounter I faced. Now, I have diverted this question to "How can I solve this problem? We need solutions. Do not blame. Doing that really helped me face my growth and embrace myself for the better days ahead. We are now in today. You have a new day, therefore, a new beginning or chapters must be embraced but not live on past experiences. We can only look back when we want to reflect to help us move forward in life.

Don't be confused about learning yesterday's lessons and focusing on past events. Yes, it is good to reflect on yesterday's activities but don't blame yourself for the mistake, c`mmon, move forward, reflect and move on.

Yesterday is already gone, and we learn the experiences of yesterday to brace with the actions we face today and in the future.

Reflect on what you want to do today. What do you want to do today? What is on your to-do list? The major things you will be doing today, write all of them down.

Work on your dreams with the action you take today not yesterday.

It's fine to celebrate success but it is more important to heed the lessons of failure.

-Bill Gates

Learn and correct the mistake.

A Mistake! Why do I have to make a wrong move? It is a Mistake.

As humans, as we are, we are bound to make mistakes or wrong moves in life. There is a popular quote I do hear people say when they make a mistake on their priorities, "every mistake is a new style", and it is mostly carried up by women. Especially, when they decide to be creative in an initiative and it goes wrong. When people laugh at them, they often say that to help them uplift their confidence levels to keep on going and not to look down on themselves. You will hear these quotes just to give the creator motivation to upgrade themselves on the artefact created. Thus, a mistake is a door for new initiatives and innovation; giving room for learning through flaws. It is mostly heard among African women.

The most important aspect of learning from our mistakes is to give us the clue to try again. Try again until you get it right. Sometimes, I engage one of the search engines when I need results. When I key in the term, the search results shows me what I want to know. I wanted to know about the .com., so, I clicked to open the search URL slug, but nothing came. I was expecting a fully operating website, but it gave me a short description, "site cannot be found." What! Let me try again, I said to myself. I tried again, same result. Then I changed the keyword and got it. This time, it didn't give me "the site cannot be found" but rather, what

I wanted. With this, it can happen in our interest areas. What are we dying for? What are our priorities? We hope to see good results come our way, but then, we realize a mistake has been committed. With the least expected encounter, we say, what is happening? We can either try again or never try again to find the exact cause of the wrong result. When you try again, it insinuates that we are eager to search for the flaws of what went wrong.

A mistake can never be corrected when you are unaware of your steps. When you are not conscious of the action you take, you just move to the wrong path. You are on a strong stand if self-awareness and change is your priority.

We change for the better. We learn new things about life, trends going on, and a lot more to grow our personal development.

> *"Do something new each day"*
>
> \- Brigitte Adofo Agyapong

Do something every day.

There is no perfect thing in pursuing success. It is a destination. If you are hoping to achieve your dreams, be eager for those dreams. Everything is possible. The dreams are big, and you want to start achieving them. Yes! you can when you believe, but one thing is for sure, you can't be out of the blue, wake up and expect your dreams to be achieved. Tiny steps, then small things, to the big achievements.

The most efficient thing to do is to use your time effectively and efficiently. Don't procrastinate. You want to achieve these dreams, but each day you procrastinate that "oh, I will start it at this time," and procrastinate again. By the time you will be self-aware, you will have a year of zero accomplishment in your action towards your dreams. Know how to use your time and don't waste time. Plan your daily itinerary towards your goals each day. At the end of the day, I need you to assess yourself, "Was I able to achieve my daily plan for today? Ensure that you don't decide on big goals or plans that you can't meet; it makes it impossible to accomplish them. Be realistic and do something new every day.

When you use your time effectively and do not waste the full plans of your goals on minor pleasantries, you will realise that each step is powerful and great because they will combine into a huge task of progress in your dreams.

"Energy is contagious: either you affect people, or you infect people."

— T. Harv Eker

Fuel your mind with YOU.

Fuel the mind with you. Don't allow the blame from others towards life to rule out the life you hope for. Energise your mind with yourself. Everyone has aspirations they wish to achieve in their lives. Why must you focus on what your friends will say about your dreams or goals before you will be fully convinced to pursue them? Since you lack the confidence to push through, you allow friends to instruct your dreams for you. You definitely know you can do it; these dreams are possible and yes! you will do it. You allow the naysayers to criticise you that this is never done in our family or society, whilst your instinct knows it is possible. Your dreams are possible no matter what. The innovation you want to create is possible no matter the obstruction. You can do it.

You have the authority and responsibility to execute and control your life. As soon as you give room for naysayers and those who judge you to come into your mind, the mind with the assistance of the thought will process their actions and words into your being and way of life. You will not be yourself anymore. Now, instead of the mind knowing you as a unique person with different competencies and abilities, it will know the naysayers' opinion of you, therefore, your life will transform into the naysayers' code. Now, your behaviour will change, and you would not be yourself anymore. You will become a whole different from the former. Fuel the mind with what you love. Accept your flaws, your challenges and your abilities. The mind is you, and therefore should be handled with care and love to flow with the commands to benefit you positively.

Developing Affirmation words for your to-do list

1. **What do you want to achieve after speaking an affirmation into your life?**
2. **How do you feel when you say that?**

How to affirm:

- Develop the willpower to do this. Be eager to execute your daily mantras.
- Prepare a list of words you strongly believe can energize you, like powerful, beautiful, and a lot more.
- Use pronouns like "I am" for positive results.
- Never use "I am" for negative emotions such as I am sad, I am horrible, etc. due to our humble servant, the subconscious mind, because it works.
- Get a journal to write down all your affirmations (powerful words, with powerful titles or affirmations)
- Exert your acceptance and belief. Add faith when you are saying it.
- Decide your schedules. Thus, you will say your affirmation in the morning or evening.
- Post your power words on your wall, where you can see them each day.
- Better still, add them to your vision board.
- Add them to google notes or calendar.

Principles are what allow you to live a life consistent with those values. Principles connect your values to your actions.

— Ray Dalio

Establish values and ethics.

When you decide to pursue your dreams or aspirations, there is one step you have to take to rule your life in order to achieve these accomplishments. When you get stuck in the journey, there are paradigms to restart and continue the ruling of your dreams, though it becomes hard when you experience such things.

Adding value to your life provides a greater height to succeed and rule life. Establish values and ethics to brand yourself. What values and virtues do you want to establish? Assess what you love and stick to it. Some of the virtues can be determination, hard work and sharing of love. These are just a few of them to mention. Why do you have to set these values? You are asking right; these are entirely important in shaping and modelling your aspiration to come true. You need principles to guide you to steer these dreams into success.

You can't achieve the big dreams you always wish for without establishing these foundations. Establish it to create a personal culture to run your life. When you do so, it becomes your habit or character. You can't achieve your dreams without being determined and persevering. These are just a few values you can set. Knowing these virtues and ethics can help you achieve those dreams. Plan on the things you love, and shun the habit that stops you from achieving them. Stick to those virtues and ethics.

The secret of your success is determined by your daily agenda

- John Maxwell

Develop your daily Mantra.

There are a lot of personal development authors, counsellors, life coaches, and psychologists who have said a lot about mantra. Mantras can be called affirmations. Setting a mantra should be part of your routine and the daily tasks you do in life. Mantra is spoken words we say to ourselves to flow the power of the words into our lives. Our words are powerful, and every command flows from our being to run in our subconscious mind. It is necessary to set and proclaim these mantras into your life each day.

Establish daily affirmations that you can develop to proclaim greatness, and let them flow through you to establish things or your priorities in life. Everything will work for your good when backed with acceptance of the words you say and if you believe in those words.

> *Let go of people who dull your shine, poison your spirit and bring you drama. Cancel your subscriptions to their issues.*
>
> -Steve Maraboli

Throw out the negativity

Don't allow negativity to rule your life. When things don't go or work well with you, think about the positive side of the situation. Don't say negative words regardless of the situation you are facing because the subconscious mind is controlled by you, and whatever you say, it will follow. By the command and acceptance of your words, surely it will come to pass. I called the subconscious mind a humble servant.

When you experience financial instability, it becomes very difficult to believe that things will turn around. Hope sometimes becomes difficult, and every effort to change the situation to the best becomes hard to do. We sometimes say words which block the turnaround of our situation because the words we say materialize with the belief we attached to them. Truly, you won't see good things regarding your finances because of your belief that it is impossible to change. When you experience sickness, you often say "this disease will turn me to death." By the humble servant, the subconscious mind will command the mind and everything around to work according to that. Due to what you said backed with belief, the disease you often claim will take you to death will exactly follow those beliefs established. Not only to sickness or financial difficulties, but it also applies to all walks of life, all areas of our life which require acceptance and faith to come to play. Throw out negativity from the mind because the day you accept the words of negativity into your life, it becomes your code of habit which governs your life. Throw them out to achieve greatness.

Dream big, start small, but most of all, start.

– Simon Sinek

Begin the Journey.

Don't wait, start the journey anyway. This journey is the path to making your dreams a reality. The most important thing is that you have decided to succeed in making this dream come true.

Begin this journey. Be strong on this decision. As far as you want to start, imposter syndrome and doubt will begin to run through your mind to stop you from believing in yourself or pause on the journey. You will get words such as "I am not worthy of this", "I don't have the necessary experience to start", and "What if I fail at this? When you start to experience these thoughts of self-judgment, it is a great thing because it proves that the instinct and the energy to start are strong, and you are on the edge to take the lead step in turning these dreams into action. Congratulations on that.

It is normal, just relax. This is a simple trick I usually do, I relax and develop a designed affirmation that suits the dream problem where the imposter is attacking. If it is writing or another endeavour, I create it according to the problem I want to solve and often tell myself that I believe I can do it and that my proposed customers or target audience are always in dire need to patronize my dreams to change their life. Try this when you experience self-sabotage (imposter syndrome), and remember that this encounter took time to develop in your conscience, then take some time to clear your mind. Do affirmation slowly whilst you allow a way to clear the imposter syndrome, and continue working on it. See it as a waiting period. Until you are fully empowered to move high, just work on it. Relax, and begin in any way you can.

Open up your senses to grab more opportunities. They are everywhere, gather and use them.

– Brigitte Adofo Agyapong

Open up your senses.

Opportunities are everywhere; so as are challenges or threats. You lost one chance of opportunity that could have changed your status to a hero a few minutes, hours or days ago. You made it slip by and finally decided that there are no opportunities near you any more. This isn't true because there are a lot more around you. Opportunities are everywhere. There are some even in your room, outside your home, on the tv and many more.

First of all, I would like to help you change the mindset that there are no more opportunities around; for you to realize and see it well. There is a need to prepare the mind so that you can create or reveal one because the initiatives I will show you require a positive and strong mindset. It is important to open a door of your senses to grab the information, to trigger the mind that this is an opportunity. With opportunity, you sense it, capture, reveal and work with it. Our senses come to play when you want to grab them. Opportunities are available for those willing to use them.

You must have the willpower to use it. With the abilities of self-aware, you will successfully grab it and start using it. Open up your senses to embrace the activities you do or the events around you. That is a massive step. Starting it afresh isn't easy, but when you can rehearse your mind on them, you just have to sit down and it will automatically trigger you. When you enter opportunities, be aware of your senses. Sometimes, I grab my opportunities via a Television show or a conversation with a friend or things around me. It all starts with one action and ends with one thing for sure. The more you use and turn opportunities into ideas and work on them, the more the mind triggers you when you enter into an opportunity zone.

When you visualize, then you materialize.

- Denis Waitley

Visualize all images.

Would you love to turn your own images into ideas? One of my favourite quotes regarding imagination is from Pablo Picasso which states that "everything you can imagine is real." I really love this quote because Mr. Pablo proves to us that the images we see in our heads whether good or bad are real. You can either believe and build upon it or never do it at all.

Imaginations help us to create ideas because these visual images combine to create one meaningful idea. Our mind has the ability to create different images that we see in our imagination to form ideas which help us to invent. Though sometimes, we see images which we hardly believe can come to pass, imaginations tell us the opposite. There are things or activities we visualize that we hardly see around us or have seen less of it around us, but imagination makes it possible. When the mind sees a collection of images from our internal and external environment, it is able to form mental images through interpretation, and further process them to help us understand the concept of the image formed. Also, after the mind has understood and fully processed them into the thought system, you can recognise and remember what you have seen in your imagination. Do you often get ideas? When you do, what do you do with it? Do you just brush it off or do you try to pen it down or record an audio so you don't forget about them? It is mostly to reciprocate this act to produce more ideas from your imagination. The reason is that the art of writing down your ideas makes the subconscious mind plays a vital role since any information moving out of the mind unto the paper or book is said out of the mouth, and the action of memorization goes back to the subconscious mind to be stored and remembered. Each time you do that, it remembers the mind to take the action to work on your ideas. It is real when you are to combine these images into ideas. Always remember this process when you think about imagination and visualizing new ideas to be used in life.

When you visualize, you generate powerful thoughts and feelings of having it now. The law of attraction then returns that reality to you, just as you saw it in your mind.

-Rhonda Byrne

Build these images into ideas.

When you are able to visualize the images you see in your mind, the brain makes it possible to interpret and process the result of the combined images. These images are then interpreted as an idea. Ideas don't come out of our minds as perfectly already made. They are raw. They come in their raw state. As an agent of idea creation, what can you do to make it appealing and applicable to the society or the environment?

The first step to follow when creating and making these ideas work is to jot them down. If you have started the habit of journaling, write down all the images the mind has produced. Combine these images and write them down as seen in your imagination. If writing is not your thing, you can pick an audio recorder or video recorder to gather the images as seen.

Then later, sketch the ideas by assessing the first surface of an ideal creation. You can ask yourself these questions. What problem are the images going to solve? What inspired me to create these images or ideas?

Research everything you have to know about the solutions you want to bring into being. Is it a product or service? Do these ideas have similar products around? There is more to researching deeply. Niche down the idea until it becomes clear. The more you get the ideas clear, the more initiatives are open to those ideas. When you are able to develop these ideas, continue to create branches of those ideas that can be developed in the future. Idea creation doesn't stop when you develop it. Always open your thought to new ideas.

Assuming you are found in a community of few libraries and bookstores and you got the idea to create a bookstore and an e-book bookstore. You have to start assessing the idea on whether to make this idea work and if it is needed for you or the society. Research more on the idea and create more unique products or services. The more you research to make the initiative clear, the more you have clearer ideas about the initiative. As you think deeper, more new niche idea areas are developed. Build ideas and dive deep into making them real and clear.

An hour of planning can save you 10 hours of doing.

- Dale Carnegie

Start Planning.

"Failing to plan is planning to fail"- Benjamin Franklin. Imagine you and your friends decided to organise a small party, can you say the party can be a success without planning? No! It is strongly needed. I believe planning is vital in making the party a success. The location, food, lighting, sound or music, gift, invitation cards and more requires planning.

After building your ideas, now what? I don't think you are going to leave the nice idea to work on its own. You need action, and for actions to move on smoothly, you will need Plans. You must start the plans on the next point after the idea creation process. What can you do to skyrocket the idea into action? Where to start and how to start depends on how your planning and organising will be. Don't just plan in your mind. Prepare a document to back the activity you do, and make it successfully executed from the feasibility studies through to the business plan and the various planning document to manage and direct the reality of the dreams.

Each time I create images and form them into ideas, I do a roadmap and a rough assessment to prepare the mind for the exact product or service I want to bring on board. Then I start feasibility studies, conduct a market study and make a business model and finally business plans. Apart from business plans, I also create various functional plans like an annual marketing plan or an operational plan. These documents are mainly used as a directional map to guide, coordinate and organise your ideas into a real-time business or venture.

These are a few planning documents to make ideas work. All the plans you will indulge in to make your dreams work require character. A character of self-discipline and a change of mindset. You can prepare all the beautiful and powerful plans filled with ground-breaking strategies to uplift your dreams into reality, but one thing that can change all these willpower strategies towards your actionable dreams is the mindset. A mindset ready for success is all you need because, with this, you will be willing to work towards everything possible to make your plans successful. One thing pivoted is, don't just plan and make all these documents without using them. Use them and make yourself subject to change. Don't wait for tomorrow. Start now.

The man who moves a mountain begins by carrying away small stones.

- Confucius

Start working.

Dreams are beautiful and nice when you create them. The energy behind when creating and drafting your dreams in your journal or notebook is a great feeling. It's amazing. The energy to start and achieve this dream was strong that I wanted to start as soon as possible. The experience was great and amazing. I asked myself some questions like How can I achieve this? Dreaming is a good thing to do in your lifespan. Dreaming big is a great thing to talk about. The most important thing for your dreams is to start working and making action to bring them to life. This requires a bold step and tenacity.

I guess you have asked yourself this; How am I going to start on this? Just start. Don't wait to be perfect or invest in all your abilities before you start working on them. Don't wait to be skilled before you work on your dreams. Work and skill up your abilities, and by the time you will realize, you will gather much experience as you train yourself on the way.

This is how I started my consulting career. I discovered my love and interest in consulting when I was working at then time Beige Savings and Loans Limited as a Sales Representative at the financial institution. My role was to increase the bank customer portfolio by bringing new clients to the firm, thus, convincing new customers to register an account with the financial institution which also requires an advisory tool to the proposed client.

As I execute my entitled duties and along, I sometimes review proposed customers' business problems and give them solutions, thus, advising them. I realised I was good with the advisory and also giving out strategies. And I also realized that my recommended solutions are working when I do client review. One Saturday, after some busy house chores, when I was reflecting on my identity and my passion, my mind took me back to the scenes on how I easily flow when it comes to advisory and how the recommended solutions also work. Then I discovered that truly consulting is part of my life and a way to impact people around me. I then asked myself, "now that I have realized consulting is my thing and I know nothing about it, how can I learn about it? Immediately, my inner self told me; invest in yourself. Find a school that can train you on it. I quickly took my mobile phone, surfed through google and typed some keywords relating to consulting training. I saw a lot of schools offering consulting training, and I visited the selected schools` premises. To my surprise, one school had branches in other African countries so I thought this was good, but when I went to the school's location, it was closed. I then picked another school from the selection I made. I visited the school and they gave me the necessary information and enquiries about the course. I later chose a school which is the Institute of Certified Business Analysts and Consultants (ICBAC) after I did a little research. I decided to be admitted after the research and started investing in my consulting career. Let the schooling begins. I began the training. Now, I am happy to say I am a consultant still learning more and more.

This is just a short story of mine to convince you that whatever your dreams are if you start working on them, they can become a reality. Working on them requires time, sacrifice, determination, hard work, and a lot of grit to make it possible.

Let's get the work of dreams to begin and continue until we reach there.

Don't give up on your dreams, or your dreams will give up on you.

– John Wooden

Believe in your dreams.

The word "believe" comes into this context when you have accepted that you can achieve your dreams. What is your priority? What do you want to achieve? Dreams can be small or big, but do you know something? Let me tell you that no matter the size of your dreams, just hope and accept that those dreams are achievable in life even in challenges. The most important thing is for your dreams to move in line with your purpose, and working in line with them requires the habit of patience and timing, thus, knowing when the time is right to start, stop or pause. This will assist you to pivot these dreams to the right destinations. Forget about the criticisms you often hear. Do you know you are the only person who knows your dreams and understands them? This is because these dreams were created out of love, and only you know who you want to be, where you want to be, and the in-depth of those dreams. No one knows the energy, the love, and how these dreams were created except you.

They will say all sorts of words to you just to stop you from working on them. "You are not worthy", "you are not perfect", and all sorts of negative words to redirect your dreams in their direction. You love your dreams right? Then it is time to believe in it and say to yourself "it is possible", and "my dreams are achievable no matter what." Say these things to yourself each day to gather the energy to uplift your mind, body, and soul. This will help you to push to higher heights in the realization of these dreams.

*You are a shining star.
Arise and shine your star.*

- Lailah Gifty Akita

Buckle up, arise and keep the fire burning.

The fire is about the energy to drive you to work. In achieving your dreams, it can be a rough path sometimes. You will encounter problems, and financial constraints might set in just to stop you from working. Mentally, you might judge yourself that I can't do it at all or even progress. These are blockages just to stop you from moving. Each one of us has his or her problems relating to dreams actualization. Events and other activities that we do or others do to us can affect these dreams.

An example is a male drug addict and dealer who got rehabbed and changed his way of life. He ceased the trade and the use of illegal drugs. The whole community in which he was located knew he was "a drug addict and a dealer." The battle of life changed him; thus, he lost his beloved wife to drug abuse. As time went by, the pain, blame and grief were all on his shoulders and later got arrested and served his punishment in prison. All these experiences convinced him that he has to change, and he did. After he was sentenced and served in the prison, he came home and took a bold step to give life a second chance by starting life afresh.

One of his dreams was to build a high school for talented children which was to enable all classes of families to receive a unified education. He successfully built the school and made the necessary documentation and legalization to licence the school. Finally, the school was licenced. Now, it was time to admit students. He started running adverts to convince parents in the community that his school is one of the best. After several weeks of advertising and all the necessary marketing strategies to make the school run, no change happened. No child was admitted into his school.

On one of the days, as he was walking through town, he heard something which broke his heart. Guess what! There were rumours in town. He heard from diverse groups conversing, and some of the words include "Have you heard a new school has been opened in town?" Another lady: Yes, "I will never send my children to a school built and owned by a criminal", they extended, "How can you plan to send your children to a criminal school?" and "do you want your children to be criminals. He was overwhelmed by the words floating in the community; thus, his dreams and the school project have become the talk of the day negatively. He wondered why the community is attacking his past, a past he doesn't want to remember anything about lest he doesn't want to return. People were judging him because they were not convinced that he can start anything good with his life. The community was just pushing him away so that his dreams can be shattered.

We have a lot of dreams and endeavours we want to embark on, but sometimes we are pushed away from pursuing them. I am proud of this man's story because he realized that he needed to change and transform his life. He had a dream and pursued it. The only problem that was hindering his progress was the people in the community who were mentally attacking him just to stop the dreams from happening.

Are you facing a similar situation like this scenario?

Don't let the hindrances you face now stop you from working on your dreams. Encourage yourself. You are going to achieve it no matter the problem you are facing. Lift the energy up and move to higher and greater grounds. Everything is possible. Keep the fire burning, continue working and don't stop.

Energise your star inside of you. Boost the drive and inspire your star for greatness and purpose.

– Brigitte Adofo Agyapong

Develop an inspiration booster.

As humans, we sometimes slip on what we want to achieve in life. We work on our dreams, but it's not every time that we get the spirit to pursue them further. We sometimes feel like giving up on our desires and what we are pursuing. The high energy which keeps us going actually declines, and we don't feel the urge to push forward any longer. The high energy gets reduced, limiting us from pursuing those dreams. The willpower to continue gets to a crush, and we feel like forgetting about those beautiful dreams we usually dreamt of and the high energy attached to them.

Due to the negative attraction we receive; the negative words and actions towards us push us to stop pursuing. There is nothing wrong when you feel like giving up. You are okay when you experience that. This happens when the pressure of life pushes you to stop, and therefore, you no longer have the desire to strive for your dreams. It is a normal process for us as humans, and the only remedy is to get words of inspiration from yourself to just rekindle the energy inside of you to a higher level. To continue pursuing, you need an inspirational booster. A booster that can motivate you to continue and develop triggers that push you going.

Look around you. What motivates you to keep working on your dreams? It can be people you have impacted; who are sharing their testimony of progress with you on how you have impacted their lives due to the execution of your dreams. It can be anything like yourself; the small progress you are seeing in your life, a motivational speaker, your religion, and many others. These boosters can increase your momentum to work again on those dreams. Sometimes, when I feel like giving up on my dreams, I just cease the process to take a week or two off to rekindle myself, think about the impact the execution of the dreams will have on people's lives and their businesses just to raise the energy high again to keep working on them.

If you are working on your dreams; be it a business person or an employee of your dream firm. Whenever you feel like giving up, just give yourself some space off work to raise the momentum high. Anything related to work should be off your head. Reflect on how you have transformed lives and the progress you have seen in your life, relax effectively to bring the energy back.

If the people around you have said something which might have discouraged you from moving, inversely turn their negative words into positive ones. See the brighter things in the dark. It can also be a booster to push you harder to work again on your dreams.

What is your booster? Discover them.

The key to successful leadership is influence, not authority.

- Kenneth Blanchard

Influence others too.

The power of influence is key in transforming dreams into reality. The main aspect of influence is to convince and persuade people around you. These are not just words but a mixture of our words and actions to influence others. It is also about impact and support for one another.

Influencing people requires service, sacrifice and integrity. We have seen that people with influence are mostly public figures or popular people in our societies. Most people often had to wait to become popular figures or known as rich men before they can start influencing others. There is no need to wait for these things to happen before you persuade other people into greatness. Your words count. Integrity and service also count. Whatever word or action you want to use to influence others, just do it. Let the word out. Don't wait.

Create urgency for people to understand whatever message you want to send across. Influence people on the things you love to do and be inspired by them. When you are able to do that, the energy in you increases because a message of influence is always backed by inspiration and interest, therefore, you give the most out of yourself to your followers or fanbase. Picking an activity you hate can't spread the word of influence.

Learn more about how to influence people around you and why the power of influence is key in assisting your dreams.

Win You: An introspective journey of finding yourself, knowing your potentials and harnessing them for greater heights and ultimate success. It can be found on the resources page. Win You has an in-depth knowledge on how to influence and persuade others.

Life is what happens when you're busy making other plans.

- John Lennon

The life is here.

Are the bellows of life hitting you hard? Hard that you want to discontinue this beautiful journey of turning dreams into reality. Are you on the edge of quitting because you are not seeing any progress or improvement as planned towards your dreams?

This is what I have for you. Don't stop yet. There is a gift I have for you, it is the word "hope." There is hope for the future. Hope manifests itself in times of situations; it shows itself strong and convinces you that you can try again. Believe and hope work together. There is the need to believe that the situation of failing in your endeavours is just a temporary thing. Have faith in every endeavour you embark on. Without it, how can you raise the energy level to keep on working? You might even refuse to embark on other aspirations when you lose hope. You will come to accept total defeat in life, which will stop you from serving your purpose on earth.

Hope is around, hovering to find, mend and uplift the broken and shattered pieces of you together by a single action of belief; so that you can keep working and pushing.

Worry is a misuse of imagination.

\- Anonymous

Pack the worry away.

We worry about what will happen in the future. We worry about how our dreams can be possible in life due to the words we hear from the external environment, such as what people around us say. "No one in this community has ever succeeded in completing this task, why do you have to pursue it? It is impossible." You are wondering whether you will fail in this endeavour because others have failed in the same dreams you want to pursue.

Worry works in line with fear. You experience fear due to worry. Are you worried that others have failed massively? Though some have lost huge capital due to the execution of the same dreams you want to pursue, pack away the worry. There is no harm in trying on your endeavour. Failure is part of the success story. As you fall, you will learn from the experience and gather the strength to keep on going. I will like to tell you this: "Worry is the misuse of imagination" – Anonymous.

It prevents you from working better towards your dreams. Let 'worry' know that you are in charge of your success, and you will succeed with your mind and body. Pack and remove worry from your life, and away from the positive result that is coming. You win, right? Win everywhere.

Nothing is impossible, the word itself says 'I'm possible.

- Audrey Hepburn

Nothing is impossible.

"This is difficult, I can't do it." "There is a lot of competition and risk in achieving this dream. It is impossible." Sure, you said it right, but I will tell you this, everything you want to do to ensure the realization of your dreams is hard and looks impossible.

Just believe you can do it. One thing you have to do now is to motivate yourself so that it can increase your willpower and push you to keep on working even if you feel like quitting because of the fear of difficulty. Embrace yourself in it.

This is what I usually do when faced with difficulties. I affirm this to myself anytime. "I am a fighter and a winner, and I will fight until the end and win." Anytime I say that, I get the energy to pursue harder, and the energy becomes stronger and pushes me to execute more.

You can try an affirmation that works for you. When you are saying affirmative words, don't just say it for saying sake, believe in the words you say.

Doubt can only be removed by action.

- Johann Wolfgana Van Goethe

Remove doubt from your being.

Doubt stops you from believing in yourself. Doubt often is classified as imposter syndrome. This type of doubt starts when you decide to pursue your dreams, and it follows you when you launch the activities of your dreams. Thus, even when you start working and people in the society start to recognize your effort and commitment to the endeavour, you will still experience doubt. Sometimes, you will get the feeling of whether the beneficiaries of your dream will like what you are executing as your dream. There is always this feeling that whispers about project perfection. "Would they like or hate it?" You also think that if my product is bad, they won't trust me again. Just relax.

All these give you the chance to demotivate or degrade yourself towards working and believing in your dreams. Through my experience with doubt, more especially, the imposter syndrome, it often comes into play when you decide to develop an action to make the dreams work. Then if you can pass through this stage by working on it, it stops, and you will not experience them in your head again until when you decide to let the world know that this is your dream and you want to execute it for the world to see, then it hits you strongly again. It influences you to think that the activities you want the world to see must be perfect and yours aren't perfect. Also, naysayers will finalize and increase the doubt because you will perceive that what you are saying inside you, thus, the doubt and what the society is saying are true.

In order to continue pursuing these dreams, you need to take action to clear the doubt. You can do that by identifying your booster or taking the decision to believe you can do it. Though it might be hard sometimes and will not be easy doing them, you just have to persevere and remember the sole reason why you want to pursue this dream. Don't rush to develop the belief at once. Develop it slowly with words of belief to build you up.

"Every day is a new opportunity to begin again. Every day is your birthday."

—Dalai Lama

Give life a fresh start, there is nothing wrong when you fail.

Wow, you made a decision! Congratulations on starting again. Though this might seem simple and easy, you made a bold step to start again. I am happy for you.

Starting again means you have reflected and realized to begin afresh. You might try again due to the lessons you have learnt.

Don't worry when friends and loved ones are moving high on their aspirations. Remember life is not a race, and everyone has his or her time when things move on smoothly for them. The most important thing is that you have accepted to rise again. A friend once told me; it is better to fail than not try at all – Ebenezer Anane. It is great you are trying again, and this time, you will gain an upper hand in experience than the fresh beginning. Just keep trying and learn more from the experience.

Building and repairing relationships are long-term investments.

– Stephen Covey

Build a relationship with others.

There have been a lot of messages about self-help. "Take full responsibility for your life because no one can do it for you." It is absolutely said right, because you are the sole person who can decide who you want to be and where you want to be. The future lies in the decision you make now, thus with yourself.

What if I told you, you need others too to help shape your life? We live in an environment where we communicate and live with people. Your success and failure sometimes depend on them. Picking the right allies can help you a lot. Building the right society of people will help shape and push you to greatness, and it serves as a strong stand to live your dream. You cannot do all things by yourself. You need the help of others too. Have you seen any business succeeding without working with people? No, whether you are a sole proprietor or a company, you need people; employees, suppliers and many others who are stakeholders. So far as people are around you, you need them.

There is a need to build a network of individuals and firms that can help push your endeavours. Picking the right ones is key because it can help you on the journey as you move on in life to build a network with others. I mostly build a network with people at conferences and seminars, social media, in fact anywhere I find myself. I draw near to them and learn more about them before finally, I will decide that these people are good to help me on my journey. "Does it mean we should pick good friends always? No, good and bad networks always help us on the success journey. The bad network sometimes helps us to learn from our mistakes and grab changes if we are self-aware of our actions. It assists us to tell a strong success story since no one is perfect. Even with a good network, you might discover bad nuts in them, so it is part of the process. What I want to say is that build the right network that can help you to grow and elevate you into greatness.

Build a network of cordial relationships with other professionals. They can be friends, family, or people you meet at conferences, forums, marketing events, parties etc. One social media which is mostly filled with professionals, investors and firms is LinkedIn. You can build strong relationships with other professionals through this platform, LinkedIn. You can also build relationships on Facebook, Instagram, Quora, YouTube, and other social media platforms.

When you found yourself at any event and wish to network with others, introduce yourself, develop relationships with them by having a chat with them, and exchange contact. After the event, try to contact them via phone call, SMS or email. As time goes on, build trust and that is it, you have built the relationship. Some relationships can help you when you found yourself on an awry path within the task of your dreams. You can also share professional ideas with the network you have built. Everyone gains when you share ideas, context and solutions to problems in life or business. Flashing back, the first time I got myself on this network endeavour as an introvert, I was on my sales job at an insurance company. Oh my God, it wasn't easy but I had to do it. I had to network to get some leads. I was already found at the event so I had to do it, though I was panting as a first-timer. Battling with my thought on these words, "I can`t do this, can this be possible?" But finally, I said, "I will do, Ooh, I breathe in.

I have to do this, that is why I am here." By the time I realised, I was having 20 lead contacts, I personally went to network with them. "Now, what do I have to do to create the bond, build the relationship, and let them register for some insurance package," I said to myself.

To my surprise, some of the leads are still friends of mine today due to networking. There is a need to build one, if you are an introvert like me, don't worry you can do it too.

> *It's very refreshing to go away and take a break, to clear your head, and just get into something else.*
>
> \- Francois Nars

Take a break.

Break time! Take a break from any task you are doing in your endeavour. You have seriously work on it. Great job! You are doing well with this endeavour. I will need you to take a break or rest small on them. Take relaxation in your neighbourhood or outside your area.

You can visit a serene environment to view the natural environment. You can take part in a family picnic, a stroll at the park, or visit the zoo, estuary, beach or anywhere outside the home that can give you a break from your activities.

Relax a little. Pick a day or days in the month or quarterly to relax. This will help to also increase your energy because you will go back to work or on your task with a fresh mind, fresh ideas and strong energy to keep on going.

Surround yourself with people who support your dreams and love the dark scars you want to hide away from the environment.

- Brigitte Adofo Agyapong

Surround yourself with people who will support your dreams.

―――――――――――――

Are you working with dream movers, or you are moving with dream drainers? The type of people you move with can determine whether your dream will go far or not.

The problem we mostly face with people is knowing them, because some work with you in disguise, but inwardly are not in support of what you love or do. Whenever you rise to improvement and draw nearer to how your dreams can come to reality, they will give you all the praise you need to let you know that you are surrounded by good people who support your dreams, but their actions will tell it all. Their actions show the opposite of it all. They are never happy with your progress. Surround yourself with people who will support your dreams. Be self-aware of things that happen around you. Don't be open to their words only but their actions too. Just be vigilant with how they behave. Assess yourself and your friends, and this will help you to decide whether you are on a good or bad path concerning the people around you. Though the bad and good are all part of the success story, be vigilant.

Open your eyes to embrace the true friend who supports you. They can support you emotionally, financially, and mentally. Wondering how to see true friends or supporters from the bad. It's easy.

"You will know them by their fruits" (Matthew 7:16). This verse makes it simple; you will see them by the fruits they yield. Thus, their character or behaviour. Remember you still need others too, but picking the right one is a good thing to do.

"If you want to go fast, go alone. If you want to go far, go together"
- African Proverb

"Fill your paper with the breathings of your heart."

– William Wordsworth

Start journaling.

You have heard a lot about journaling. Journals are this and that. Yes, a lot of people are saying start journaling. There is no problem when you do that. More professionals who are into the power of the mind such as psychologists, psychotherapists, Physiotherapists, counsellors, coaches, authors, and other professionals have said a lot about the habit of journaling, and it is a good thing to do.

Journaling is the art of writing down your priorities and events in your life in a notebook or journal. Research says it helps promote our mental and emotional well-being.

Since you are on the urge of achieving your dreams. You will need an idea journal, mood-tracking journal, project journal, gratitude journal, meditation journal, prayer journal and many more journals that can be used to record your activities in life.

You can also record your journals on your phones or tablets on a digital planner, or make audio of anything you want to journal about.

A mindset is needed when you want to start this habit. What do you want to achieve after each day of journaling? What do you want to gain from this exercise? Is it going to help you change your lifestyle or reach a new horizon? It all depends on the mindset to start and continue until it becomes part of your life.

Don't just write down your activities inside a journal or notebook, but track and use them in your life. Cross-check the activities if they are good to continue with the habit of writing, and if they are bad, find a way to stop. It serves as a guide to reflect on your life and helps you to identify who you are and where you want to be. Some of the users of journals use an emotional release journal to dish out all the hurtful feelings inside them that interrupt their dreams because of the harboured pain. A journal helps you to release them all.

Do journaling routinely. Pick a time in the day that can help you. Opt for days that can help you to keep up with your routine and honour them. See the habit as part of your life. I have my routine concerning this. Each time, I ensure to keep them up, and if I don't meet them, I ensure to change the time and date to suit my schedule.

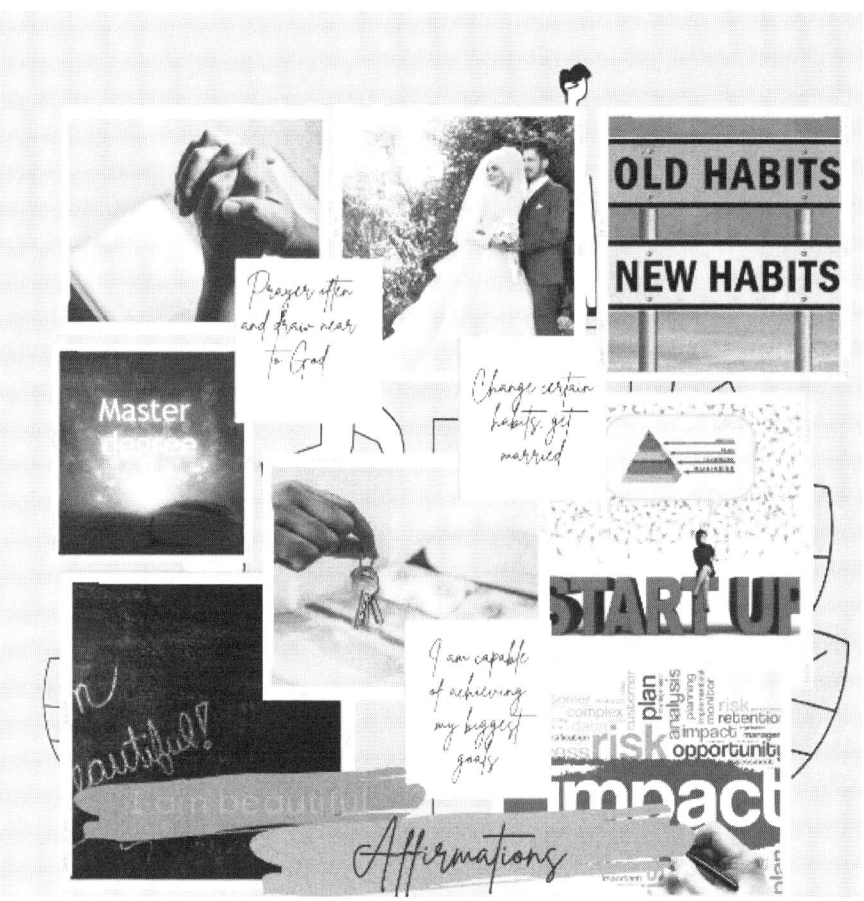

Figure 1- Sample of a vision board inside a goal setting journal

People with passion will change the world.

- Steve Jobs

The passion is yours, use it.

Each one of us has passion in us, or we have the interest to work and make our dreams a reality. It is yours! You need to know your passion, thus, your interest area and develop a desire to work with it or utilize it. You might be wondering why people say "work with your passion or find your passion." Yes! you are on the right path. You are not only finding your passion but rather, you have to follow and work with it.

An activity you pursue in life with passion provides plenty of goodies into your life because you will embark on what you love and will continue to love it. And as you work on it, it will yield the result you least expected. The heartbreaks will force you to stop, but due to the burning desire (passion) for the activity, you won't have room to give up. And even if you do, your mind will still be on it.

With passion, you move in line with your purpose in life. The exact purpose of your existence. Don't stress yourself if you can't find it. The words I have for you is to relax and find it, and never compare yourself with others when things are not moving accordingly for you because it will influence you to go and pick areas that bore you. The passion is yours, find it and use it. Don't think about anything that hinders you. Think about the interest areas that project your happiness.

To fall in love with yourself is the first secret to happiness.

- Robert Marley

Love yourself.

Have you started pursuing your dreams? If Yes, it means you want to succeed with them. Great on this action. But to continue, you need to love what you do. The feeling and the interest are essential for your progress. It shows how much you love that activity. As far as you have shown interest in this dream, it means you will give the maximum love and attention to whatever you are doing to be able to work on this task.

If you have exhibited some dreams but don't love the activities involved in realizing them, how can you continue to pursue them? It is not good because when challenges hit you hard, the energy to move on becomes very slim since you don't love your dreams and the interest areas.

If you don't love your dreams, it means you might be forced to move in line with your purpose.

How will you feel when you try your possible best to realize your dreams and later decides to give up because you have lost interest in it? All the practices that made it perfect and exceptional, you have decided to lay them down out of your life. Then suddenly, a surprise hits you hard. A work you thought wasn't receiving enough accolades from people, thus, no one ever praising you that they were cool and could solve their problems, people criticizing you that it wasn't good. Then one day, people around you started to receive it with great joy, bringing out great testimonies on how your work is helping them and that they are beautiful. What will you do? Will you give up or put more energy into it?

This experience is like a lady who was into crochet bag weaving. She started it as a hobby because she loved it and made her happy any time she did it. Also, it serves as an escape from the pain she was going through. Each day, she practices it and gets down when the final product doesn't look beautiful and classy. Since she loves it, she always encourages herself to continue weaving because it brings joy into her heart. Guess what? Some of her friends and even people whom she tried to sell the bags to mock her, saying things like "they are ugly just like you", "who told you people will love it" and all sorts of negative things just to discourage her. Sometimes, she feels like giving up but then remembers why she started and continues. One day, a prospective client showed interest in it and finally patronized it. Each time she would try to give up, that is when people would bring out their testimony of how good she is or how beautiful her product is. Whenever they say these words, it gives her the energy to pursue harder and tries to remind herself to push more.

This is to tell you that your love for your dreams can take you far. Life is neither smooth nor rough. You will experience both the bad and the good times when pursuing your passion. How can you stand the test of time when you don't love what you do? It is very easy to give up because of the lack of love for the actions you take towards your dreams. When you experience setbacks and feels like stopping, your interest in whatever you are doing can fade faster due to the unloving attitude towards your dreams. It leads to low willpower to continue. You have to move in line with your purpose and love what you do. Seek what you love that brings you happiness. Own your dreams and love every activity you do about them.

Appreciate every step you take and love who you are and who you have become.

- Brigitte Adofo Agyapong

Appreciate these steps.

Before an athlete will run 100 metres or 1500 metres, it requires a step. A step at a time will slowly take you to a destination. Now, you have started pursuing your dreams with actions. These actions are steps which will take you to greatness. It will lead you to success.

More times, we want to achieve great results before we can be happy about what we do. Appreciate every step you take to empower yourself through the journey of greatness and possibilities. Love the little progress you have shown.

Assuming you are a project team leader on a project to solve uncleanliness in the environment or the neighbourhood. You and your team are planning to make an initiative that will convert waste into profitable clothing fibre. The team decided to create a machine to make the initiative possible. Each time the team put in an effort, they fail, and when this happens, you humiliate, shout, and disgrace your team members on why each step to build the machine has failed. The best thing to do for your team is to appreciate whatever steps they have added in making the initiative possible. Praise your team members with words like "you are doing well, add this and that, let's try to create value in this area or that area." As you try this, your team will be exposed to clues to solve the problem and make it successful, and finally, execute to solve the problem of uncleanness in the environment. With appreciation, by the time you realise you have created the machine and will be at the stage of testing because you made the team aware of their mistakes, and it has finally yielded results.

Gratitude helps you to grow and expand; gratitude brings joy and laughter into your life and into the lives of all those around you.

– Eileen Caddy

Be grateful.

If I would guess, you are asking why being grateful comes into this circle about dreams realization. Yes, it comes into the context because being grateful can make and unmake your dreams a reality.

Dreams achievement requires emotions too. Since you live and work with people, you will need them to push you higher to originate yourself from your inner self. I mean, you have feelings too.

Being grateful is all about self-love resulting in minimal blame, criticism, comparison, jealousy, greed and a whole lot more. To pursue these things, you have to be kind to yourself, love whatever you do, and be happy for who you are because a fallen mindset with low self-esteem and low self-love can't push you anywhere. You will experience low energies to work on your dreams, low willpower and desire to execute more, pushing harder will not be part of your life anthem because you are unkind to yourself and ungrateful to who you are.

Be thankful for each day of your life and your progress. Execute more to yield more on this journey.

Success is liking yourself, liking what you do and liking how you do it.

- Maya Angelou

You Stopped your passion!

Why have you stopped pursuing your passion? I know you are progressing in this passion. Why did you stop?

If I have to guess or wonder, this is because you have stopped believing in yourself due to the words you heard from your friends, colleagues, and family members. Their words echo so hard in your mind that it has convinced you to stop, right? Or is it because you have lost the desire to continue pursuing them since the dreams are not yielding results as planned? You have spent several years on these dreams, but the result is nothing to speak about so you have given up on it. You bid farewell to these wonderful dreams. You are right about your decision to quit on your dreams or your passion. It is normal when you assert that you will not continue again. One thing I can share with you today is that just give yourself some time, don't rush, and close your ears to others who are flourishing on the same path as yours. You started together and now your allies are flourishing and progressing in their endeavours. You have asked yourself a series of judgmental questions and now planning to give up. You say to yourself, "maybe this is not for me."

Okay! I don't know what led to what you are experiencing. But whatever the cause, it is related to the decline of your love towards this dream. I will tell you one thing. Dreams do come true. Everything is possible. If you believe and trust that you can do it, you will surely do it. It is just a matter of time.

There are times and seasons for everything. You are in the waiting period, just be content with the waiting period. Don't stop. When your time comes, you will see how beautiful you have become because you have mastered your challenges.

A smile is happiness you'll find right under your nose.

-Tom Wilson

Just smile.

Smile and be happy. I think you can't fly on sadness to move dreams. You will need positive emotions to push you to work. Be happy with the situation you are in now. Situations and trials are all part of success.

These are passers-by. They will pass by when you accept that you can overcome them to succeed. If you allow bad encounters to take possession of your mind, they will consume your emotions and move them according to these encounters. Thus, it will pave a way for negative emotions to rule your life. Be happy and redefine your happiness. Don't allow money to define your happiness. Meaning, you shouldn't only be happy when you have money. What if you run out of money for some time? Does it mean you will be unhappy as far as you don't have it? Be happy even in these challenges.

> *If you don't like something, change it. If you can't change it, change your attitude. Don't complain.*
>
> -Maya Angelou

The complains are enough, stop!

Most of the time, when things are not going our way, we tend to complain about every bit of what is going on around us. We complain too much about every action of ours and others that we have become complaint gurus. It has become our behaviour since we do it each day. It is very annoying when you have friends who complain about anything each time. It becomes frustrating and pitiful at the same time. Since you have complainers around you, it is relatable when you also complain a lot. Complaints also pave way for you to sell your ideas to people who are not supposed to know. It is best to work in silence and keep your mouth shut.

The whole cause of complaints in most things around us comes from comparison. We love to compare. We love to compare ourselves with others. Especially, when we realize we started the same action of which we must progress but see no change. We then complain to express our worries on the matter. Don't allow comparison to hit your head, live to love what you do.

Remember, each one of us is unique in our own way. Time will tell. There are seasons and reasons for everything. Each season comes with lessons to be learned. Learn to be competent with whatever you have set in your mind. Just keep on working and going.

One can choose to go back toward safety or forward toward growth. Growth must be chosen again and again; fear must be overcome again and again.

- Abraham Maslow

Give yourself the chance to grow.

Self-growth is like growing a seed. A farmer sows a seed in a seed container kept on a balcony, waters it and provides the seed with the needed sunshine. To make it sprout and get the minimal sunshine it needs, the farmer places the seed in the window on the balcony. The farmer ensures that the seed is properly taken care of, and watches it as it sprouts. The seed starts to show a green leaf, it is properly taken care of as it increases in height and beautifully grows. When it's transfer time, the farmer then transfers the garden plant to a field. The plant is transferred to a field for it to grow well into a tree in order to yield fruits. But after replanting, it is left at the mercy of the harsh weather condition. When it is raining, it falls on the plant, the same as the sunshine. Also, it is left at the mercy of the weeds and thorns to attack its growth. For proper care of this plant to grow into a big tree and yield results, the farmer has to take absolute care of it and clear the weeds and the thorns around it. Protect the plant from diseases that might attack it.

This scenario represents us. Our challenges and our caretakers (parents, guardians, or loved ones). When we were little, all our worries, needs and challenges fell on the shoulders of our parents, guardians and some loved ones. Now that we are adults, all our worries, needs, and challenges have been pushed from our parents or guardians to us. As adults, we have to take full responsibility for our lives. We have to take care of our dreams and goals and learn to handle our challenges and scars. The harsh weather condition we face is similar to how the plant is released into the open space just to grow well, and that same environment can help us grow and yield results. The harsh weather conditions can be anything which hinders us from growing. In the same scenario, the grower, thus the farmer has all the right to protect and prepare the plant to grow and yield results by taking absolute care of the plant. To protect the plant against diseases, weeds and thorns. As a farmer of your dreams or aspirations, it is your full responsibility to protect your dreams from challenges that will stop them from materializing in life. It is never going to be smooth. It is either you uproot the weeds from hurting your plant or you allow the weeds to take charge of your plant or the farm. Imagine if the farmer didn't decide to stop the weeds or thorns from harming the plant, there wouldn't be any fruit to yield. These are similar to our challenges, it is either you face them or leave them to take charge of your life. Our growth is backed by challenges, so don't think that when you face challenges in the early stages of your dream realization and fight to triumph over them, that is all. I am here to tell you that as you move on in life with your aspirations, more and bigger ones are yet to come. As you learn and master your weaknesses, you will increase your strength to grow better and have more courage to face the problems you encounter along the way.

The seed will never grow well without the challenges.

We all can grow in different forms. The various ways we grow as individuals are never the same. What the experienced ones face to grow is vastly different from the inexperienced ones. Don't compare your level of growth with others because you are two different lovely individuals with competencies and flaws.

Personal growth involves spiritual, mental, emotional, financial and social growth. What is your priority? How do you want to grow in the personal development phase? Don't stop yourself from growing. The time to grow is here.

All you need to say is simply 'Yes' or 'No'.

-Matthew 5:17 NIV

Be firm on your decision.

You made a good decision in buying this book to motivate and keep you going on your dreams.

When we are too clinched to friends or loved ones, they sometimes control our decision. Thinking straight is a strong stand in decision-making. People allow their loved ones to decide for them, leaving behind their own decision. When they are close to them, they can't take the right decision for their life. It is like they are being spoon-fed. Whether the final decisions or opinions suggested by loved ones are good or bad, they just take and apply them according to how they were said to them.

If you fall into this dilemma, you need to change and be firm in your decision. You need the preparedness and readiness to take charge of your life.

Is your surface filled with people who push you to make bad decisions? Don't worry because from this day forth you are no longer going to listen to their discouragement. It is important to know that you have the sole responsibility to either accept their discouragement or reject it. The results mount on us; whether good or bad, so the decision is ours.

They that will not be counselled, cannot be helped. If you do not hear reason, she will rap you on the knuckles.

-Benjamin Franklin

Open up your ears and heart for advice.

Self-help is a good thing because it helps you to understand the essence of taking advice and taking full charge of your life. The effect will come to you but not anyone else. In the nutshell, you are the sole person who will act. It has helped a lot of people and there is no doubt about it. There has been a misconception of self-help that you don't need the help of others to shape your life. "Oh, I am self-aware, no one has to advise me." I think with that, then there is no need to listen to opinions from experts, attend motivational conferences and seminars, or read books, even this book. The best point is that you want to change your life and add up value to it that is why you have been experiencing some of the things I have mentioned.

You will indeed need professionals and loved ones to advise you when you fall on the wrong path or if you want to grow your energy to keep the desire up. You will need a piece of advice to keep you running towards your dreams and soar high in them. We all don't have the same experience and expertise.

Everyone has his or her level of experience and distinct skills. These skills defer. When professionals and loved ones approach you, it may be because they have seen a mistake on your path and due to their love for your dreams, they want to help you to succeed.

Open up your ears, heart and self to receive advice. If you want to grow spiritually, physically, mentally, emotionally and financially, you will need them as your backbone. Use your intuition to clinch to them.

Learn to trust the journey, even when you do not understand it.

- Lolly Daskal

Life is a journey, not a race.

I have said a lot regarding the message "life is a journey" in most of my messages. Yes, life can never be a race. It is not a fast-and-furious movie. It is a journey that takes time to pass through.

Someone can start life successfully today and fail tomorrow, another person can fail today and succeed in the future. It doesn't mean one of the scenarios is better than the other. Thus, a person who failed in the beginning, cannot be termed as a failure whiles the other as successful. It does not work that way. They are all enjoying the same success. The only difference is how they will enjoy the success.

It is called a success zone. When you enter the zone, whether you like it or not, you will succeed because of your decision that failure is never going to dominate your life, but rather you want to succeed and overcome your challenges, and surely, you will do it.

When you fall, instead of feeling ashamed over the fall, do this: tell yourself that "this is not a race, and I will rise above all odds because I am stronger and more powerful even in these challenges." "Though life has hit me hard and made it difficult for me to rise, I will rise and fight until I win. Even when I win, I will win and win until the end." Gather the courage and start again. Don't worry when naysayers ridicule you with words like "see, your friend is already gone on the success ladder and you are now about to start over, you can never reach there." Loved ones will ridicule and say all sorts of words to keep you sited where you are so that you can't move. They do this to instil in you habits such as blaming yourself, comparing yourself with others and many more that will move you to develop the wrong mindset.

There is nothing wrong when you start again. This time you may have learnt the lessons that resulted in the fall so you are going to move and move faster.

Succeeding in life is not a smooth path, it is mixed with wonderful experiences to learn from. Sometimes you just want to stop and feel reluctant about your dreams. Other times too, the energy is high that you keep up with work and feel nothing can stop you from excelling. It is life. Nothing is perfect and the task is in your hands to make it good.

You can relax and study, gather the momentum and continue, but don't stop. One thing for you is to engage in the dream you have passion for. This is because passion keeps you going when you feel like stopping and encourages you to move ahead.

"Live life step by step."

- Brigitte Adofo Agyapong

See challenges as a step to victory.

Before I realized my purpose, when I encountered problems, I often say to myself "why these challenges? I can't do it"

When I realized my purpose, I discovered my sense to see threats as opportunities. This sense always triggers me when I sense things around me that are challenges and opportunities. That does not mean I see opportunities in all my encounters. No, but this is because I have prepared my mind. Therefore, my sense grabs the information and allows the mind to do the process and then I get notified.

Opportunities are always around. There are few times opportunities come as real opportunities. Most of the time, they come as challenges or threats. All you have to do is to identify the problems, and with your fundamental rights, you will be prone to solutions to solve the problems.

Spread love everywhere you go. Let no one ever come to you without leaving happier.

- Mother Teresa.

Share love too.

We demonstrate love through the words we say and the actions we take. There is much joy in demonstrating love towards one another because when you do so, you can feel peace within you for a long time. There is an urge of expressing kindness to yourself and other people around which makes you happy.

You can inculcate the habits and attitude of love in your loved ones. This can be done when you share your knowledge with others for them to also learn from your experience. Sometimes, it is very difficult to share your story with people around you, especially with the regret attached when you don't feel comfortable sharing them, but for love, it conquers all those doubts. This helps you to decide that the love behind the story you share can also impact and transform lives.

When you share your knowledge, you bring out your painful experiences for the world to hear, and it serves as a therapeutic encounter for you to release those painful expressions from within. It brings peace of mind to you.

The more you share the knowledge you know, the more knowledge and wisdom you gain.

Experts say, "one way you can learn is to share with others how to do it as you did it." This act can be classified as sharing love. As you show people how you did it, in a process, you learn new things from your act of service. Are you thinking about losing all your knowledge to others through a single act? Don't be shaken, you have more to grab. You rather gain more knowledge and your experience becomes great. Don't be discouraged to do this because of bad experiences and encounters. Nothing good to lose.

I always say that sharing love is an art of kindness. Don't focus on the result you will gain from the love you're expressing, such that the person you are expressing the love to, will reciprocate the same thing to you and others. I will say, just look at the good impact coming to the beneficiary's life such as happiness, peace of mind, and many more benefit relating to transformation.

This art can be noted as a task of exhibiting your purpose in life

Be clear about your goal but be flexible about the process of achieving it.

- Brian Tracy

Be flexible.

Flexibility comes into play when we are setting goals and developing systems that can ensure that they are achieved. We often make our goals and plans rigid. We make them rigid to the extent that it prevents us from meeting them. We have attached ourselves fiercely to these goals that by all means, we must achieve them, even if our capabilities can't reach there.

In the end, we feel embarrassed and don't want to work on it again. We give up. Making your goals flexible is a good thing to do to achieve your goals and plans.

The first step to take in preparing the mind for your dream actualization is through setting goals and working on them. These goals must be flexible. Make sure you set goals you can meet. It is good to set big goals, but you can effectively and efficiently meet them when you set short goals for a short timeline, not long goals for a short timeline. Let's say you decided to set a goal to become a professor in one year. But currently, you don't have the resources to do so within a year. In the end, you will realize that it's impossible to meet that goal. This is because the goals you set were big for a short time needs based on your capabilities.

Pick big goals, then break them into semi-goals under the same goals spreading them to each year. Then develop a road map.

Relieve yourself from the stress, set goals now.

- Brigitte Adofo Agyapong

Set goals.

In the previous message, we spoke about making our goals flexible and setting the right goals for the right time frame. Now, this is what we have to do to prepare goals for our lives. In order to set things straight and develop goals for your life, there is a need to reflect on the goals set and achieve them in the stipulated year. Bringing this one, my mind goes back to the new year's resolution. With this, it is not only a new year resolution but the entire year. It is necessary to reflect on the goals you were able to achieve in the previous years; the mistakes you did which prevented you from achieving them, and the work-in-progress goals. You will write it down in your notepad and reflect on each goal. How you did it and the next goals.

You can also push goals that you couldn't achieve but want to achieve into the following year. Write them down and add them to the following year's goals.

Each month, assess your progress on the goals you set for year one. Imagine you want to start a business and you make yearly goals to start, in fact, this year. With this, you will assess yourself from month one to month 12, your performance toward this goal each year. As to whether you are making effort to launch it and finally start it.

At the end of each month, you need to assess them. Develop a new height you want to reach; new goals you want to achieve. What are some of the goals you want to achieve in addition to the work-in-progress goals achieved? You have to identify them. Now write your goals down in a journal or notebook.

Develop systems to make it work. Develop a road map for your plans and add up your plan B. I often call it 'What if or Alternative plans.' Anything can happen to stop our dreams and action, but when you have these plans, you are still sorted on achieving your goals and plans and know when to execute them. In two-three decades, the banking system was tedious to send money to other countries, but now we have a lot of fintech firms making money transfers easy and convenient. This is a scenario which indicates that our plans must go with time. Though there are times to execute certain plans, that does not mean we should merely plan for our goals but rather put the best plans that suit the best time.

I have simple steps to assist you to set and implement your goals.

Materials you will need for this:-
- ☐ Journal or a notebook
- ☐ Pens
- ☐ Colourful pens
- ☐ Sticky notes

Steps
- ☐ Reflect on your previous goals.
- ☐ Take your journal and write down all your goals for the year.
- ☐ Before you do that, ask yourself why you have chosen this goal, if there are any hindrances that can stop you and how you can implement it.
- ☐ Write your final decision down.
- ☐ Break down your actionable plans.
- ☐ Break them down into monthly tasks (determine the number of goals you want to achieve in each month. Do it according to how you can do it and the time frame or schedule. Don't force yourself.
- ☐ Draw a line representation of each task for each year.
- ☐ Access yourself each month and find the necessary recommendations to move forward.
- ☐ Head to the Get materials page to download resources to guide you.

Staining your heart with grudges and resentment won't help. Clean it up.

- Brigitte Adofo Agyapong

Be open, don't harbour pain in you.

Most of us fall short when it comes to harbouring pains inside us. We do this each time we feel that someone has hurt us. You can't accept the fact that someone has hurt you with their words and action whilst you demonstrate love and trust to them. You expected a strong bond with them, but they eventually broke your trust and love.

You are setting your emotions at work. Emotions are big for your success. We use them every day, whether in sadness, happiness, anger, fury or many other emotions we express. You pass through tragedies leading to emotional trauma which makes you shelter a whole lot of painful thoughts and expressions. If you are asked to explain or tell about a painful event you have encountered, you will say it without leaving a mark to speak about. You will remember every scene that happened because you can't forget about the encounter and exposure. It hurts and is very hard to forget, especially, when you reflect on the relationship, love, trust and the end betrayal. You don't want to forget and let it go.

I understand how much you are hurt, but it is time to let it go off your mind and heart because you have to live in peace with yourself; your inner being, achieve your dreams and live in harmony with others. Be open, don't close yourself when you feel like gushing out your feelings. Don't hold your emotions in because when you do that, it can compound the emotions in your being and your thought will always remind you of the picture and how it happened. You then focus on that to hurt yourself.

In most African societies and cultures, when someone is in grief for the loss of a loved one, it is better to cry out all your pain to be free from the agony. When you want to harbour pain inside you with a mindset of achieving your dreams, this combination doesn't work perfectly. If you want to turn your dreams into reality, there is the need to have a perfect match of good emotions; because holding in pain will stop your mind from seeing clearly the imagination and thoughts to support your aspirations.

Therefore, for the success of this journey, learn how to manage your pain, fears, and hurts. Don't hold on to a situation where emotions will control you to move in the wrong direction. Release your mood in a mood or emotional mastery journal, it serves as a boost to strengthening your moods.

Be strong and courageous. Do not be afraid or terrified because of them, for the Lord your God goes with you; he will never leave you nor forsake you.

- Deuteronomy 31:6

Add Prayer too.

We need to add spiritual aspects or applications to our lives when it comes to the realization of our dreams. We master and grow our mental, emotional, and physical beings leaving the spiritual aspect aside.

Add prayer too. Prayer gives you a space to talk to God. He knows our heart desires and will show us the way. The book of Proverbs 16 : 3 (ESV) says, commit your work to the Lord, and your plans will be established. With every dream you want to pursue, pray to God to show you the way. He can show you the way through dreams, and the knowledge to apply to what you want to pursue and how to do it. Also, a prayer to God can lead you through the challenges and can pave way for more blessings.

The fear of the Lord is the beginning of wisdom. Pray always to get the direction to lead you on the journey of life. You know I have said a lot about the race of life, and that this journey is undefined. Prayer can give you strength backed by faith, and with belief, you will move greater and stronger. Don't leave prayer out of the action when you want to achieve your purpose and dreams in life. Pray each time.

"Reflect on your life as to whether what you see regarding life achievement is the real person you want to be."

- Brigitte Adofo Agyapong

Develop a step Model to Succeed.

Draft a Step model to assist you to succeed in life. This book has a lot about the motivation you will need to embark on the dream actualization journey. Here is a model I have developed to assist you to define success and work on it. I have tried it too.

S - Specify your success code

We have heard a lot more about success. Success is this and that. I have one question for you. I guess you have heard about successful people and their acts. What is success to you? To be able to work well in this model, what is success to you? Reflect on your life as to whether what you see regarding life achievement is the real dude you want to be. People choose a mansion or a pool of wealth as their success whiles others choose happiness. Do you have to choose between these two? And if you have to, what is your choice?

Have a sit and reflect on what you really want in life, and how you want your success to be. This assessment is to help you on the road to developing your code to success. Specify it, make it clear and write it in a notebook or hang it on a wall, maybe as part of your vision board for your life. The success of others can't be your success. I don't want you to regret your success when you finally make a choice and start to pursue it. And finally, when you fully achieve it, then you will realize that "Ah, the choice I made for success was never my thing, let me develop another one." I don't want you to waste your life and later realize that in all your life you have made a bad choice and lived a regretful life. I don't want that.

Instinctively, reflect and specify what you want.

T- Tackle your fear

Whenever you plan to start an action leading you to achieve your dreams, and also set some questions that contemplate that you can't be successful and that you are going to fail, these questions create a threat to you to never touch this dream of yours. Before you can fully succeed, you need to work on controlling this fear. It came in just to stop you from moving. Tackle the fear, work on the fear, and empower the mind to succeed. Develop some positive vibes to slowly curb the fear in you. If the fear generator is people around you, it is better to cut off that relationship because the more they get closer to you, they will never allow you to move. Train your mind; empower the mind with strong affirmation, and start the habit of self-love. Find a way to tackle the fear and succeed in life.

E- Energize the inner self

Discover your strength and weakness. This will help you to know when to act and when to retreat. This is all about knowing yourself, your identity, and being self-aware in everything you do. Since you know yourself, when weakness strikes, you will know what to do to make the internal environment okay. Energize yourself with the training of the mind, develop mantras to guide your day, journalize each time and throw away all emotions that hurt from your being. Develop breathing exercises to guide and shape your inner matter, and exercise the body since an energized body is a strong mind. The energizing component people use to uplift their bodies and inner self can't be the same as yours. Know what works for you and stick to it. Sometimes you have to try other initiatives also, like sharing love and knowledge, it also paves the way for energizing the inner child.

P- Prepare a plan of where you will be, and set discipline straight.

Prepare and develop a working plan on how you want to succeed. Meaning, you are going to develop the habit of goal-setting. Develop a working plan to launch your success code. Set discipline straight to start.

Clinch to others who can help you move forward on the elevation ladder. Either you learn from them, or they learn from you. It's a two-way affair.

- Brigitte Adofo Agyapong

Clinch yourself to other professionals.

You can't succeed all by yourself. You need to learn from others. Most successful men and women we see around have a bunch of mentors and advisers they look up to. They study under them and learn from them. Pick a discipline you want to embark on and choose your mentors from the area you have chosen.

In my consulting career, I chose someone who is into management consulting and in the area of organisational development and strategy to be able to study under him. Even after a tenure of learning from him, I still see him as my advisor regarding my consulting career. I still go to him to give me tips and advice regarding what I do in my role as a management consultant. Anytime I face a baffling experience in the industry and work, I just contact him and pour out my worries or requests to him. He is always ready to help me out with all my problems and the steps I need to succeed in the career path I have chosen.

Don't just choose any mentors. Niche down the area you want to master or develop and pick mentors relating to that. You will need expert advice to still shape yourself when you are found on the success path. You will still need their bits of advice and tips to push you through.

In my debut book, 'Win You: An introspective Journey of finding yourself, knowing your potentials and harnessing them for greater heights and ultimate success,' I said a lot more about how to find mentors and how to invest in yourself and time. I would like you to learn more on this particular topic from 'Win You', and advance more on clinching to the right persons. Visit the resources page of this book, and discover how to get hold of it.

It is not the answer that enlightens, but the question.

- Eugene Ionesco

Learn to ask questions.

Do you know it is good to ask questions? Yes, there is nothing bad about you asking yourself some questions or seeking answers from people you trust, or even clearing your thought when you are uncertain and needs clarification on certain things around you. Doing this the right way is the best. Are you wondering what is the right way? Let me show you this, but before that, let me give a clearer note on asking questions.

Some do ask themselves a lot of questions or others too much on one particular problem which makes them complaining gurus to others and themselves. It is like they aren't satisfied with life.

For things to be clearer for you and your life, there is the need to ask questions about your challenges, feelings and dreams. We use the questions to clear or reflect on our being as to whether we are moving on the right path or not. Questions are daringly important. Most seminar and training programmes have a bunch of questions to ask you when you want to start a training or seminar. They are known as learning outcomes. They are usually asked to open the participants' minds to the training outcomes and the impact on their lives. When you want to know the truth about certain things in life such as finding your purpose, seeking happiness, and growing a positive mindset, always ask questions. When sales volume is not producing as anticipated by CEOs, management and directors, there is a lot more to say about the beginning and the end with your ability to ask questions. There is the need to ask questions to get answers and then make a final decision on our plans.

The habit of asking questions is a positive stand to reflect on the experiences you see today, in the past, or even in the future. This serves as an avenue to reflect and learn about the progress in your life.

Learn to ask questions when you reflect, examine, and seek the truth about your life and anything you show interest in. Don't refrain because you think people will say you like asking questions or people often say to you, it is bad. Though it can be boring and frustrating sometimes, I think you have to do it in the right way and reduce the level of judgemental questions which can harm you or others, like planning and framing questions, blaming questions or ridiculing questions to others just to mock them. Please don't try that.

People who know me know that Brigitte likes asking questions which is good sometimes because it makes you get a clearer understanding of certain things around you since perception can misinform sometimes. It is good, but it becomes boring sometimes if the questions to make stuff clear are misinterpreted into a different thing. I got the habit of asking questions to people around me, even clients from my consulting journey due to the act of diagnosing to ditch our clients' needs. A good consultant or coach always asks questions, but the right ones. For me to succeed in this career path, there was a need to ask questions to clarify things on what a client really wants; to execute solutions. One time, a client told me to help him with his task, and I started asking him questions about the task project. He told me, Brigitte, why are you asking so many questions? Just do the work. I told him, How can I execute the work without getting a clear picture of the project or the task I am about to do? I want to understand everything. I want to learn. I don't want to move to and fro in the process of doing the task well whilst you are here to explain things to me. You have to give me a clearer picture. He smile and gave me the right information and the work was executed as it should.

Another scenario was when a client came to me to help her with business strategies. When I started asking questions, She said, why Brigitte? I thought your duty is to give me strategies that will work for me. I replied calmly, I need to ask you some questions to get a clear image of the problem you are facing and do some research on it in order to recommend effective solutions for you.

These scenarios are not to take you through my role as a consultant but to bring you the common idea that asking questions is good and can give you an upper hand in understanding, not to fall victim to misinterpretation or misunderstanding of information.

Learn to ask questions to reflect and examine the things going on in your life. As an achiever who wants to move high on the ladder of greatness, questions can help you to learn from past events in your life.

> *You can measure opportunity with the same yardstick that measures the risk involved. They go together.*
>
> – Earl Nightingale

Take risks.

Believing and working on our dreams is one of the big risks we take in our journey of possibilities and greatness. This is because, with dreams, you believe, anticipate and do all of the things you think can turn your dream into reality, knowing that you can succeed or fail. You believe things will get better even if it does not seem they will.

We take risks all the time. We take risks in our careers, dream businesses, relationships, marriages, and many others.

Most app developers develop apps they believe will work now and in the future. They undertake different processes before it goes live for users to download and use. Passing through idea development, idea validation, creation, testing and so many other processes they do just to see a fully running app.

They make the necessary provision just to make it run, even though they don't know what will happen in the future. They strongly have faith in the app. They believe it will work for a long time. This is the risk they embark on because anything can happen.

We make our aspirations run just like how these developers do. You are eager, you believe and trust in your capabilities and your success, and then suddenly, things don't work as planned. Are you going to stop pursuing these aspirations? Or you are going to take the risk and move forward with your dreams? Well, it all depends on your strength to fight the challenges till the end because it isn't going to be smooth. You need to take the risk to work on them.

Using the app developers' scenario as an example, sometimes the apps they develop and work hard on get struck on the road. Things don't work as planned. They do all the processes to make it successful and pilot it, but as time goes on, customers' tastes change, causing a shift in or slow usage of the app. It is the sole responsibility of the developers to make it work again by researching to add changes and updates to sustain the app in the market.

As humans with imperfections, we will experience risk on our way to the realization of our dreams which shouldn't stop us, but rather, we will do the opposite, thus, stopping the risk. Though it can vanish at once, take time to flush it away.

Taking risks and controlling them makes us stronger. It opens our abilities and capabilities to do great things which we can't do when we are in our comfort zone. You only do them when you are in the risk stage. We kick them off, then becomes stronger, making us optimistic persons.

Take up the risk and fulfil your dreams.

Taking risks

This activity will help you identify your risks and know how to control them. I will need you to pick a notebook and a pen or pencil. Answer these questions in your notebook sincerely and introspectively.

- What are your aspirations?
- What are your goals?
- Do you face hindrances towards your aspirations?
- How will you tackle these hindrances?
- Are you going to need some help?
- If you were to advise your younger self, what will be the key advice on taking a risk?

There is always room in your life for thinking bigger, pushing limits and imagining the impossible.

– Tony Robbins

Think Big.

There is a difference between thinking big and dreaming big. When it comes to dreaming big, is all about wishing big but by thinking big, you inject yourself with ideas, thoughts, perceptions and judgments on how big you want your life to be and act on them. "They are both similar." Yes! you are right. If you are guessing that they all have the ability to do great things, keep note of this, before you can dream big, you will need thought or thinking to do that. When ideas are generated in our thought system, it is interpreted to be understood and be part of us with the assistance of our memory system which reminds us to work on our dreams, and finally take the bold step toward them.

Thinking about big things is enough said a lot because the power of the subconscious comes into play when we establish those priorities for the humble servant, the subconscious mind to follow, and then the mind will follow since we have established it to follow. Routinely, it becomes aware of the priority and then moves to the conscious mind that we are known for thinking big. We start to establish goals and take action before we can achieve them due to the power of manifestation. Since there is power in our thought, words, acceptance and faith, we start to practice them which leads to the unconscious mind. Now, we don't need the support of the conscious and subconscious mind to push us to be aware and unaware of ourselves. We don't need the conscious mind to practice the habit or our way of thinking big because now, it has become part of our life. You think big all the time.

"Motivation gets you going, but discipline keeps you growing."

— John C. Maxwell

Set Discipline Straight, and Build boundaries around yourself.

Sometimes, we get distracted from the task we have designed for our lives. You have dreams, right? You have set your goals and prepared the implementation plan ready to kick start. You are doing everything in your possible best to make your dreams successful. Everything was working perfectly, then something struck you to stop or pause, and the inner voice sounds like, "is this endeavour really for me?" Can I do this project?" "Will it actually work?" You start judging yourself forgetting all the efforts you have invested in this project or endeavour you have in mind to make your dream materialize. This scenario is telling us one thing, a distraction to stop us.

Guess what, it is never going to be perfect. You will encounter distractions just to make you stop, think, and judge whether this dream and idea is really a thing for you. The first step is to identify the distraction which is stopping you from moving or any other thing that is preventing you from implementing your action plans. Be free, don't be rigid with yourself. Prepare your mind that challenges will make you stronger and are bound to happen. Be aware of your actions and the effects of the environment's actions towards your life. Confidently tackle these distractions.

I know what you are thinking. Brigitte, I have done my possible best to stop the major distractions but these distractions attack me all the time. Let me tell you this. There is a need to find these distractions and tackle them by understanding yourself well and knowing your strength and weakness relating to how you relate with people and yourself. If the distractions are words people say to your face or say to hurt you, how do you manage them? Do you sit deep to fight back? Or you just ignore them and move on. How does it affect you? Have you considered the in-depth of words brought out from the mouth to confuse feelings? Who knows, maybe he or she is acting according to the hurt received, so decided to return the hurtful words to you. Don't let anyone discourage you from moving by indulging in the habit of negative judgment leading to blame which will compel you to stop moving. Track this distraction and reduce the intimate contact with the person causing the distraction. If your habit can cause distraction, put a stop to it. Don't force yourself. Work on it slowly because habits are developed in stages. Therefore, to put a stop to that, you need to assess yourself and examine the reward and goal you have gained or lost due to your habit and action. There are a lot of distractions fighting us from moving.

Before boundaries can be profitable, develop the virtues or values you have in life and stick to them by preparing the mind to accept changes and start to implement each value you have on board. It will be best if you start journaling on this, and read it each morning and evening. Also, you can get cardboard and write your virtues and values on the wall, add pictures and text, and remember to mark them with colours that resonate with you. Each day, ask yourself this, How will I achieve these values? Have I started implementing them? Now, what is stopping me?

Rule your life by utilizing goal setting and measuring goals. You are bound to set these disciplines to start and develop boundaries around you because you have a timeline to meet, and due to that, you know what you want in the next number of years.

Act now, and set your discipline right.

Wrap up: Dream bigger and higher.

I do like writing as much as listening to music and singing the melodies that attract me to the song. When I decided to write this book, this came to mind and would like to share it "When you dream, dream big as big as the ocean." – Ryan Shupe.

Yes, dream all along. We have beautiful dreams, what are your dreams? Do you love it? How big it is? Dream big, as big as the ocean, so big as you can. You are the sole person who understands how big your dreams are. You are the only person who loves your dreams. Don't wait for someone to tell you, "hey my friend, your dreams are so big." People will not understand your dreams unless they see them materialising. There are only a few people who see how big your dreams are. No one knows how big you want to be, except yourself.

Be you, dream and work. The messages here are to motivate and inspire you to keep working on them. Be eager for these dreams. The main purpose is to inspire and motivate you to continue working or even start. Sometimes, you will feel like stopping. This piece serves as a booster to gear up your energy. Don't stop and even if you do, remember why you started and always work and move to make it a success.

Everything needs your support. Devote your body to always support these beautiful dreams if you know they are for you.

I want to see you elevate to greatness because we are moving together to greatness.

Don't forget to share with friends, family and other loved ones the message of this book to assist them in living their dreams of greatness.

"Successful people interbreed wisdom, knowledge and love"- Brigitte Adofo Agyapong.

Impact and succeed.

Enjoy your success and elevate.

Brigitte Adofo Agyapong

Note to you, my dear reader.

I am glad in doing this! You grabbed my book! I would like to use this space to thank you for buying and reading this book. I appreciate your interest in my books and the message I send across each time. Holy grail! You read my sixth book! I can't say enough to thank you. I appreciate your support and love.

My number one motivation is to see you read my books and be motivated and inspired to achieve your dreams too. As an advocate of purpose and dreams actualization, I believe our dreams can be achieved no matter what, that is the sole reason I wrote this book, to boost your energy level up and to motivate you to keep on doing what you love doing. Sometimes, we do greatly want to achieve our dreams but feel we have to give up at some point in life because the high energy and inspiration we started with in the beginning, is off, it's low, and we need a booster to keep our fire burning and energy up. I am glad you have read this book and has impacted your life too. I hope you like it.

My request to you is that as you have read this book, don't leave the fruit hanging, use and practice it. Help others in need too. Join me as we spread the message of hope, possibilities and fulfilment in the minds and hearts of people who need our care and love through our words and actions. Help me spread this message of impact around the world to help motivate, inspire, and elevate others too. I believe when you practice and share the words inside this book, you will impact one individual which is a nation.

Spread the knowledge you have acquired from this book, impact nations and transform generations.

Always remember this "Successful people interbreed wisdom, knowledge and love."

Enjoy and impact.

Brigitte Adofo Agyapong

Bibliographies

Chadwick Bossman's motivational speech https://www.youtube.com/watch?v=DoA-a-g2o4g

Usain Bolt Success Story https://www.youtube.com/watch?v=QL5mCN-TTBs

Brian Tracy, (2010), Decide upon more definite purpose, Goals.

Brigitte Adofo Agyapong, (2021), The Power of the mind, Win You: An introspective journey of finding yourself, knowing your potentials and harnessing them for greater heights and ultimate success.

Richard Templar, (2010) Learn to ask questions, Rules of Life.

Proverbs 16: 3 on Prayer

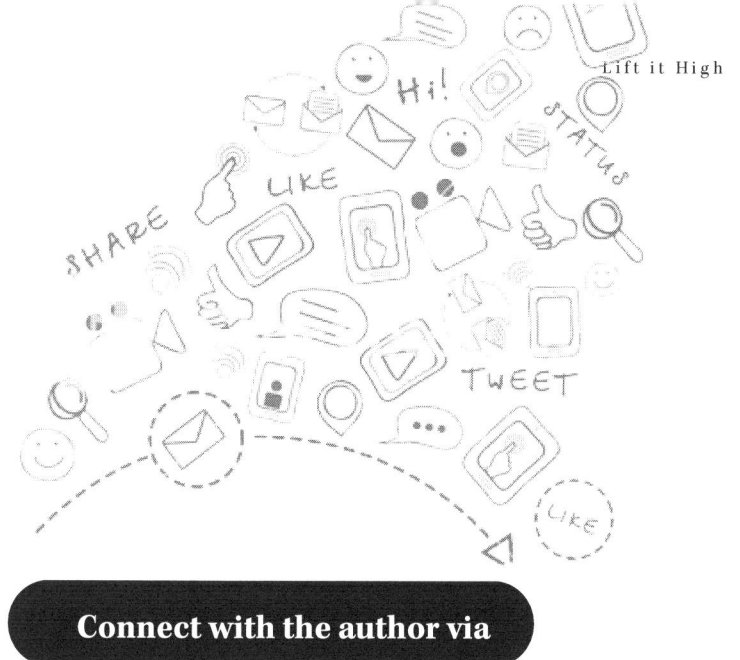

Connect with the author via

Instagram: www.instagram.com/brigitteauthor/

Facebook: www.facebook.com/brigitteauthor/

Bookbub: www.bookbub.com/author/brigitteagyapong

Goodreads: www.goodreads.com/brigitteauthor/

Pinterest: www.pinterest.com/brigitteauthor/

Value added segment

ENROL IN THESE ONLINE COURSES

I am happy doing it. I would like to see you grow. Therefore, I created a course to help you out.

With this, I have prepared a digital or online course to help you

- ✓ Visualize your ideas
- ✓ Create an idea that works for you
- ✓ Goal setting
- ✓ How to scale your business and many more

Sign up to upgrade your mind on how to build an idea and convert it into a business/initiative via this link:

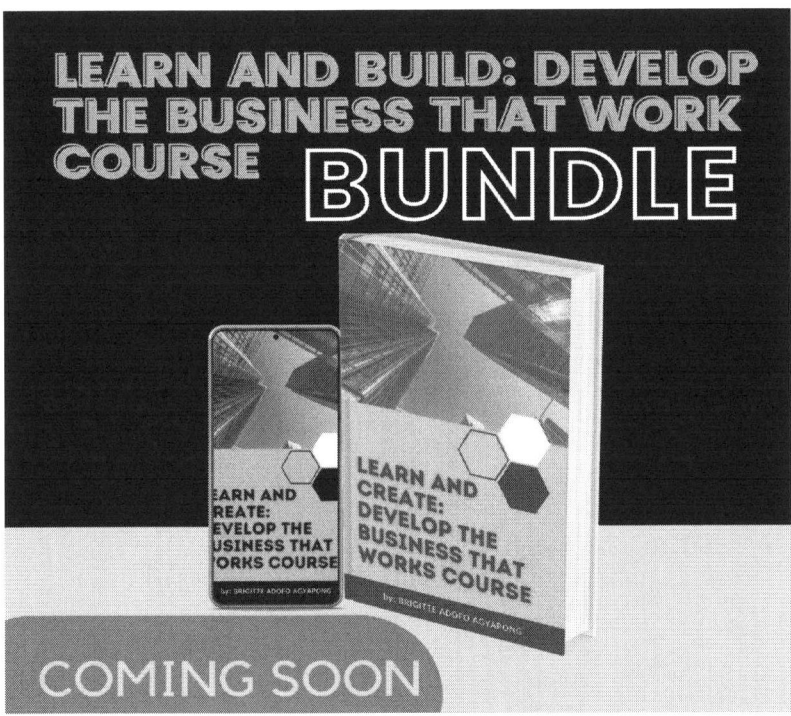

Learn more: https://www.brigitteaagyapongwrites.com/courses/

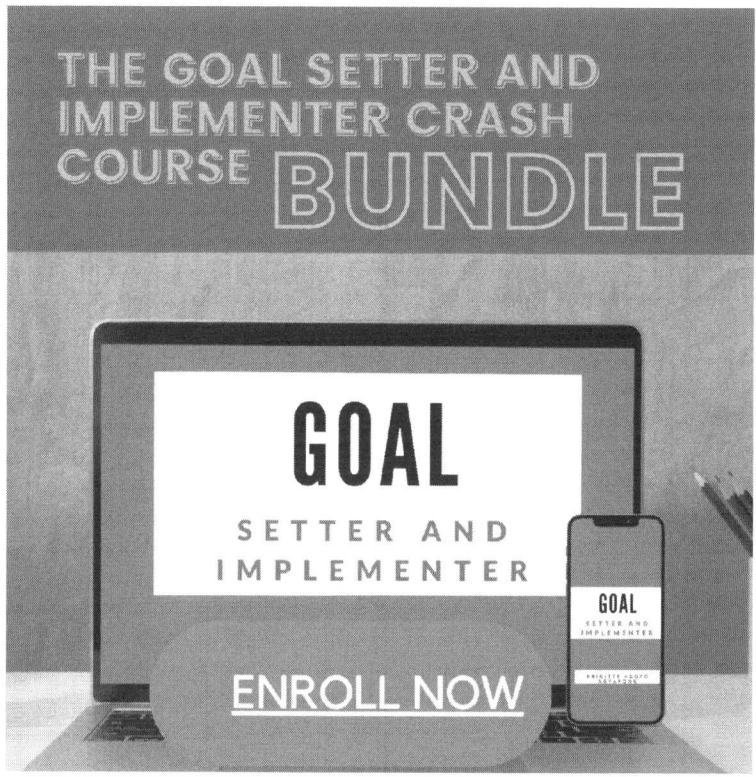

Goal Setter and Implementer course will help in the following

- ✓ Develop a good mindset to start and complete your goals
- ✓ Clear boundaries
- ✓ Implement your goals.

Enrol via www.brigitteaagyapongwrites.com/courses/

Get FREE GUIDE AND WORKABLES

Resources to download for free include:-

- A 30-day goal-setting workable
- Find your accountability partner workable

All these resources are available on my website: www.brigitteaagyapongwrites.com/resources/

Join the Community

I hope you enjoyed this book. It would be great if you write a review on the retailer platform on which the book was bought. This will assist other readers to get hold of the book and assist them to lift their energy up too. I can't wait to receive a review from you.

Also, if you experience a change or impact due to this book, kindly direct mail on any of my social media platforms to tell me more about how the book is assisting you in your Endeavour, I will personally thank you. Or send an email via: contactus@brigitteaagyapongwrites.com I will love to receive it.

Help share the word

Spread the word about this book either on a post or story, on where you are reading and how the book is helping you on Instagram. Tag me @brigitteauthor and #liftithighbook #brigitteadofoagyapongbooks

Subscribe to receive newsletters by the author via: www.brigitteaagyapongwrites.com/mailing-list/

Get a free eBook on the rules of happiness, by signing in to www.brigitteaagyapongwrites.com/rules-of-happiness

Get the Step Model cheat sheet via www.brigitteaagyapongwrites.com/resources

Subscribe to Elevate with Brigitte Podcast to learn new things about yourself, empower the mind and elevate your business.

Subscribe via: www.brigitteaagyapongwrites.com/podcast/

Also available on Spotify, TuneIn, Amazon Music, Audible, Pocket Cast, and overcast.

Other Books

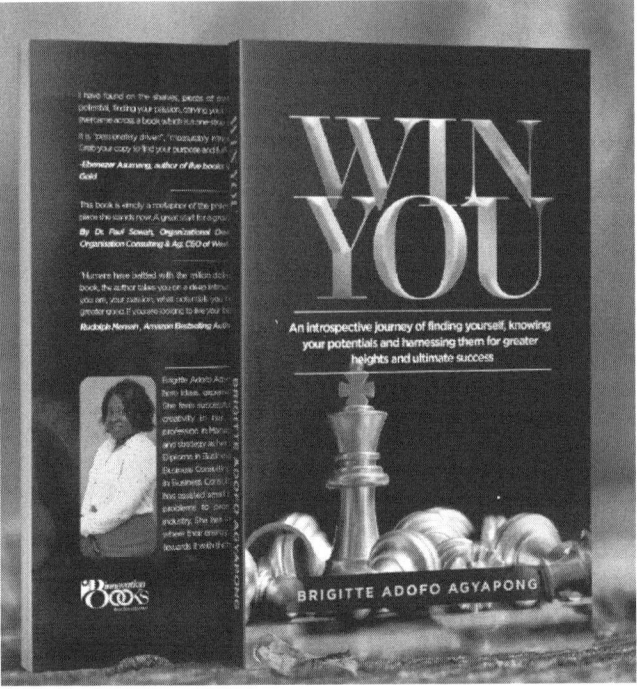

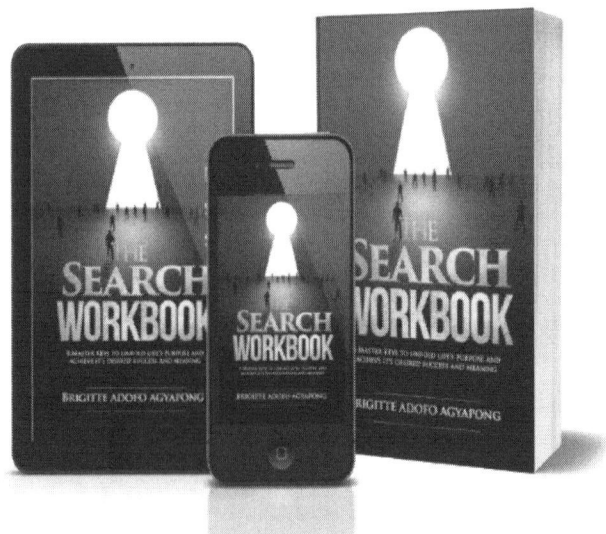

Visit www.brigitteaagyapongwrites.com/books/

Other packages for you

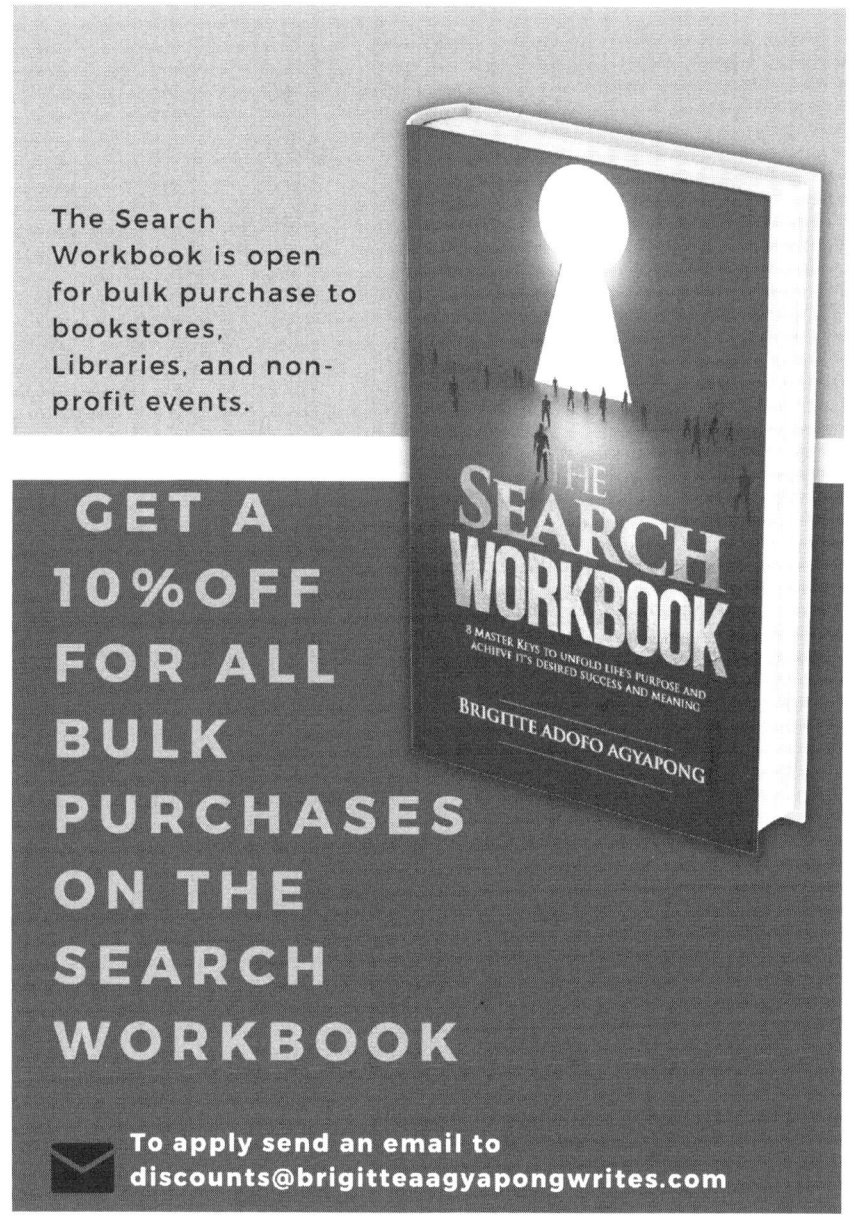

Buy all three copies of these books and get a discount of 15 %

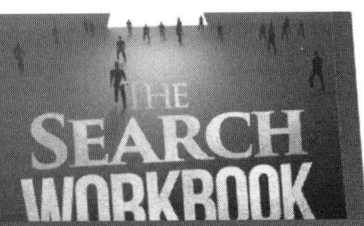

The perfect match to Win Yourself

Looking for the perfect resouces to win yourself and then the success you want?

Grab these books if you want to win yourself and others too; discover purpose, win yourself and circumstances around

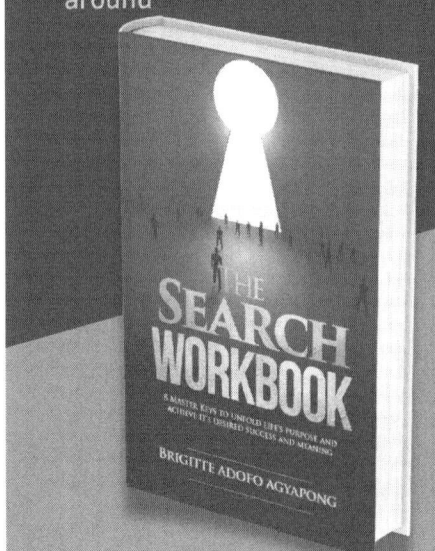
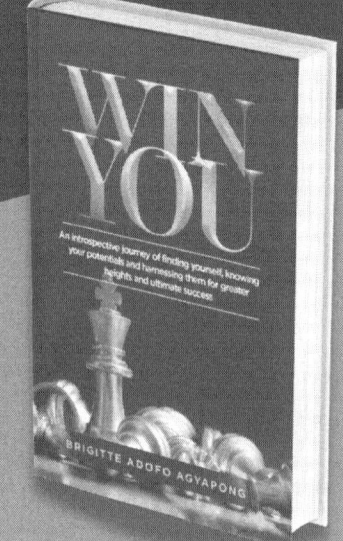

Made in the USA
Columbia, SC
20 May 2024

34958307R00112